Essentials of Reptiles

A Guide for Practitioners

An Update to
A Practitioner's Guide to
Reptilian Husbandry and Care

Thomas Huntington Boyer, DVM
The Pet Hospital of Penasquitos
San Diego, California

AAHA PRESS

Essentials of Reptiles
A Guide for Practitioners

An Update to *A Practitioner's Guide to Reptilian Husbandry and Care*

Many thanks to the AAHA Press Editorial Advisory Board:

AAHA Press
12575 W. Bayaud Avenue
Lakewood, Colorado 80228

Cover Illustration by Julie Porter

ISBN 0-941451-65-8

This book is dedicated to those individuals who have taught me so much about reptiles: Stephen L. Barten, DVM, Donal M. Boyer, Frederic L. Frye, DVM, MS, FRSM, Elliott R. Jacobson, DVM, PhD, DACZM, and Douglas R. Mader, MS, DVM, DABVP (SA). Their work is greateley appreciated. Thanks to Roger J. Klingenburg, DVM, and Scott J. Stahl, DVM, DABVP (Avian), for peer review, and to my wife, Lilia, for all her help.

Contents

Introduction

Since the publication of the first edition of this book, *A Practitioner's Guide to Reptilian Husbandry and Care,*[1] veterinary care for reptiles has surged forward. Reptile medicine now has a larger knowledge base that is rapidly evolving, in the same manner that its close cousin, avian medicine, has evolved over the past 10 years. Many factors are responsible for this. Undoubtedly the most important has been the ever increasing interest in reptiles and amphibians as pets, which has provided an economic incentive for veterinarians to gain proficiency in reptiles. Coupled with this has been a wide interest in long-term maintenance and breeding. Reptiles that were once rare, or thought to be difficult to maintain, are now bred regularly by less experienced herpetoculturists. The public has increasingly turned to veterinarians for advice, and large numbers of veterinarians have taken an active interest in reptiles. The Association of Reptilian and Amphibian Veterinarians was founded in 1991 and now lists well over a thousand members worldwide. Most large continuing education meetings for veterinarians now offer information on reptiles. Conservation of reptiles has never been more important, resulting in an increased need for veterinary involvement.

The veterinarian is often less experienced in captive care of reptiles than the owner of the reptile. This puts the veterinarian in a difficult position, because the majority of problems seen in veterinary practice result from poor husbandry. Compounding this difficulty is the fact that veterinarians receive little formal training in reptilian medicine. However, the veterinarians' background and training in medicine help them to learn quickly and borrow principles from other areas of medicine. Accordingly, this book will focus first on husbandry and then explore problems common to the most frequent presenting groups of reptiles. Additional formulary and anesthesia sections round out a sound introduction to this fascinating area of veterinary medicine. This is by no means a thorough review; the reader is referred to the following veterinary texts for more information.

Several textbooks have been published in the past few years. Undoubtedly, the most comprehensive has been the multiauthored text *Reptile Medicine and Surgery.*[2] This text has a wealth of information and is the current state-of-the-art reference. No one practicing on reptiles should be without it. Other recent texts include *The Biology, Husbandry, and Health Care of Reptiles,*[3] *A Veterinary Guide to the Parasites of Reptiles,* Volume 1, *Protozoa,*[4] *Reptile Clinician's Handbook: A Compact Clinical and Surgical Reference,*[5] *Self-Assessment Color Review of Reptiles and Amphibians,*[6] *Veterinary Management of Tortoises and Turtles,*[7] *Common Reptile Diseases and Treatment,*[8] *What's Wrong with My Snake?,*[9] and *A Color Atlas of Diseases of the Crocodile.*[10] Publication of *Amphibian Medicine and Captive Husbandry*[11] is anticipated for 1998.

Many other references are worth mentioning. By far the most informative is the great two-volume work *Biomedical and Surgical Aspects of Captive Reptile Husbandry,* 2nd edition.[12] The first edition is also still useful.[13] Another outstanding text is the *Manual of Reptiles* published by the British Small Animal Veterinary Association with multiple authors.[14] The two-volume set *Diseases of the Reptilia*[15] and *A Practical Guide for Feeding Captive Reptiles*[16] are also very good. Several older, but certainly worthwhile, texts focus on reptilian diseases. They are *The Principal Diseases of Lower Vertebrates: Diseases of Amphibians and Diseases of Reptiles,*[17] *Veterinary Biology and Medicine of Captive Amphibians and Reptiles,*[18] *Diseases of Amphibians and Reptiles,*[19] *The Bacterial Diseases of Reptiles; Their Epidemiology, Control, Diagnosis and Treatment,*[20] and *A Review of the Diseases and Treatments of Captive Turtles.*[21] Chapters are devoted to reptiles in several texts including *Diseases of Exotic Animals,*[22] *Zoo and Wild Animal Medicine,* 2nd edition and *Current Therapy,*[23] *Exotic Animals,*[24] *Manual of Exotic Pets*[25] (now into the 3rd edition),

Laboratory Animal Medicine,[26] *Exotic Animal Medicine in Practice,* Volume 1,[27] *Saunders Manual of Small Animal Practice,*[28] *Color Atlas of Comparative Veterinary Hematology,*[29] *Atlas of Diagnostic Radiology of Exotic Pets,*[30] *Reproductive Biology and Diseases of Captive Reptiles,*[31] and the *Merck Veterinary Manual,* 6th, 7th, or 8th edition.[32] *Current Veterinary Therapy*[33] usually has articles on veterinary care of reptiles and amphibians.

Several anatomy manuals are useful including *Laboratory Anatomy of the Iguana,*[34] *Laboratory Anatomy of the Turtle,*[35] *Laboratory Anatomy of the Alligator,*[36] *Laboratory Anatomy of Necturus,*[37] *Laboratory Anatomy of the Frog,*[38] and *The Anatomy of the Bull Frog.*[39] The two-volume *Life of Reptiles*[40] and the multivolume *Biology of the Reptilia*[41] are loaded with information and illustrations that can entrance this veterinarian for days. Several good references on reptiles and amphibians are *The Encyclopedia of Reptiles and Amphibians,*[42] *Reptiles and Amphibians,*[43] and *Grizmek's Animal Life Encyclopedias,* Volume 5, *Fishes II and Amphibia,* Volume 6, *Reptiles.*[44]

Several veterinary publications regularly have articles on reptiles, including the *Journal of Zoo and Wildlife Medicine*, annual proceedings of the American Association of Zoo Veterinarians (contact the AAZV, 810 East 10th Street, Lawrence, KS 66044) *Seminars in Avian and Exotic Pet Medicine* (contact W.B. Saunders Co., Periodicals Department, 6277 Sea Harbor Drive, Orlando, FL 32887-4800), the *Veterinary Clinics of North America: Exotic Pet Practice* (contact W.B. Saunders Co., Periodicals Department, 6277 Sea Harbor Drive, Orlando, FL 32887-4800), *Journal of the American Veterinary Association*, the *Veterinary Record*, and the *Compendium on Continuing Education for the Practicing Veterinarian.* For the reader seriously interested in reptilian and amphibian medicine, consider joining the Association of Reptilian and Amphibian Veterinarians (ARAV). Membership benefits include a membership directory, proceedings of its annual conference, and the quarterly *Bulletin of the ARAV.* For more information contact the ARAV at PO Box 605, Chester Heights, PA 19017.

The Chicago Herpetological Society's (CHS's) *Care in Captivity: Husbandry Techniques for Amphibians and Reptiles*[45] is also recommended reading and is included with CHS membership (contact CHS, 2001 North Clark Street, Chicago, IL 60614). *The Care of Reptiles and Amphibians in Captivity,* revised 2nd edition[46] is also good reading. Advanced Vivarium Systems Inc. (10728 Prospect Ave., Suite G, Santee, CA 92071-4558) publishes a plethora of good, affordable husbandry texts on reptiles and amphibians that are recommended for veterinarians and clients alike. Those texts are referenced in each species-specific chapter. The International Herpetological Symposium published some 16 volumes from their annual conference that contain a wealth of husbandry data. Likewise, the Northern California Herpetological Society, the British Herpetological Society,[47–50] and the International Symposium on Turtles and Tortoises published a series of proceeding from their various symposia on care and breeding of reptiles, which are also loaded with information. Many of these can be obtained through reptile book dealers (such as Zoo Book Sales, PO Box 405, Lanesboro, MN 55949-0405). There are many excellent magazines devoted to reptiles and amphibians, most of which are available in pet stores with an interest in reptiles. Specific useful references are also noted in each chapter. Some of the best lay magazines include *The Vivarium*, the official publication of the American Federation of Herpetoculturists (PO Box 300067, Escondido, CA 92030-0067), *Reptiles Magazine* (PO Box 58700, Boulder, CO 80322-8700), *Reptile and Amphibian Magazine* (1168 Route 61 Highway S., Pottsville, PA 17901-9219), *Reptilian Magazine* (22 Firs Close, Hazlemere, High Wycombe, Bucks, HP15 7TF, England), and *Reptilia* (published in three languages in Europe). Numerous herp societies and organizations are worth joining. Some of the more prominent publications include the *Chameleon Information Network* (13419 Appalachian Way, San Diego, CA 92129), *Chelonian Conservation and Biology*

(Chelonian Research Foundation, 168 Goodrich Street, Lunenburg, MA 01462), Chicago Herpetological Society (previously listed), *Copeia* (American Society of Ichthyologists and Herpetologists, Florida State Museum, University of Florida, Gainesville, FL 32611), *Dactylus* (International Gecko Society, PO Box 370423, San Diego, CA 92137-0423), *Herpetologica* (Herpetologists League, Section of Amphibians and Reptiles, Carnigie Museum of Natural History, 4400 Forbes Avenue, Pittsburgh, PA 15213), *Herpetological Natural History* (International Herpetological Symposium Inc., 361 Van Winkle Avenue, Hawthorne, NJ 07506), *Iguana Times* (International Iguana Society Inc., c/o William Hayes, PhD, Department of Biology, Southern College, Collegedale, TN 37315), New York Herpetological Society (PO Box 1245, Grand Central Station, New York, NY 10163-1245), National Turtle and Tortoise Society (PO Box 66935, Phoenix, AZ 85082-6935), New York Turtle and Tortoise Society (PO Box 878, Orange, NJ 07051-0878), Northern California Herpetological Society (PO Box 1363, Davis, CA 95617), Notes from the Northern Ohio Association of Herpetologists (Department of Biology, Case Western Reserve University, Cleveland, OH 44106), Society for the Study of Amphibians and Reptiles (which publishes *Herpetological Review* and the *Journal of Herpetology,* PO Box 626, Hays, KS 67601-0626), and *Varanix, The Varanid Information Network* (Varanews, 8726D South Sepulveda Bl., No. 243, Los Angeles, CA 90045). Astute veterinarians may also join and support their local herpetological societies.[51] See Barten[52] for more information on publications mentioned in this and other sections.

1

General Information

Several topics are important with respect to all groups of reptiles. Accordingly, this chapter will cover basics of temperature, humidity, cage accessories, ultraviolet lights, incubation of eggs, salmonellosis, and quarantine of reptiles.

Temperature

Reptiles are ectotherms, which means they are dependent on external environmental temperature to maintain their own body temperature. They differ in this respect from endothermic mammals and birds, whose primary source of body heat is internal. Reptiles have lower metabolic rates than mammals or birds; consequently, reptiles produce much less metabolic heat and thus depend on their environment to maintain their own body temperature. Reptiles also lack elaborate insulation structures, such as feathers or fur, which makes them further dependent on environmental temperatures. Terms such as cold blooded and poikilothermic (variable body temperature) are no longer in vogue. This is because many reptiles behaviorally maintain body temperatures that are higher than those of mammals and within a narrow preferred optimum range that is not as variable as previously thought.[53] Reptiles maintain their preferred body temperature (PBT) behaviorally by modifying their access to external heat sources. A few giant species seem to generate greater internal body heat, but this is much more the exception than the norm. Thus it is important to provide temperature gradients, either horizontal or vertical, within the captive environment so that the reptile can select its own preferred optimum temperature zone (POTZ). Adequate ambient temperature, localized warm areas for basking, and cooler areas allow the reptile to select its own POTZ. Most species are adapted to a drop in nighttime temperatures. The POTZ varies between species, but a good range for most temperate reptiles is 75 to 85°F (24 to 29°C). Tropical species prefer even warmer environments. Some diurnal desert lizard species prefer to be very warm, 95 to 105°F (35 to 40.5°C). Water temperatures for aquatic turtles and crocodilians should be 75 to 82°F (24 to 28°C). Submersible aquarium heaters are usually required for aquatic species because water temperatures tend to be much cooler than air temperatures. Amphibians prefer it slightly cooler, from 70 to 80°F (21 to 27°C), although some tropical frogs tolerate warmer conditions. Remember that these are only guidelines. It is best to determine the preferred optimal temperature zone for each given species.

In general, sick reptiles should be kept at the upper end of their POTZ to maximize the immune response. When in doubt, the cage should be warmed from a low of 75°F (24°C) at night, to a high of 85 to 90°F (29 to 32°C) during the day, with localized hot spots. Temperatures less than the PBT lower the reptile's metabolic rate, which decreases food digestion, depresses the immune system, and is often the underlying cause of illness or anorexia in reptiles.

Owners often fail to provide the PBT for their reptile. Important queries when taking the history of reptiles are "What is the cage temperature range during the day and night?" "How hot does the basking area get?" "Do you have a thermometer in place to monitor temperature?" and "How is heat provided?" The only way to be sure of cage temperature is to use a thermometer. After many years of checking temperatures, the author has found guesswork to be unreliable and dangerous. Insist that owners purchase a thermometer. Digital, minimum–maximum, indoor–outdoor thermometers are available from many electronics stores and reptile products catalogs for a reasonable price. These are better than simple thermometers for two reasons. First, minimum–maximum thermometers record the temperature extremes, so one has a better idea of the true temperature range during the heat of the day, as well as during the chill of late night. Also, the twin temperature probes of the indoor–outdoor thermometer allows one to monitor temperature zones in different areas of the cage or even under water.

Another important aspect of ectothermy is that reptiles have much less compensatory ability to tolerate hyperthermia. Overheating quickly kills reptiles. Glass or plastic aquariums should never be placed in direct sunlight without shade, because lethal temperatures may be rapidly reached. Most veterinarians working with reptiles have received tragic phone calls from reptile owners who put the aquarium outside for "just five or ten minutes" only to return and find a dead reptile. As a vivid example, consider the sidewinder, *Crotalus cerastes*, which survives in some of the hottest environments on the planet (including Death Valley, CA). Klauber[54] reported that sidewinders died within 10 to 15 minutes when restricted to full sunlight in a natural habitat. When one observer simply removed a bush under which a sidewinder was thermoregulating, it became "stiff as if cooked" and died in 11 minutes.[54] Smaller reptiles obviously reach lethal maximum temperatures faster than larger conspecifics.

Also be aware that reptiles are attracted to heat sources and, for reasons that are not well understood, will burn themselves if given the opportunity to bask on, under, or around heat sources. Anything too hot to rest your hand on comfortably is definitely too hot for reptiles. Heat sources are safer outside the cage and should be used within cages with caution. The following are common methods of keeping reptiles warm in the hospital or home, listed in approximate order of preference:

> **Space heaters**—Warm the entire room or a small closet. Make sure the heater does not overheat the room (temperatures above 100°F [38°C] are rapidly lethal for many species). A backup thermostat that will turn off the heater at high temperatures is highly recommended. Room temperatures between 75 and 90°F (24 and 32°C) during the

day, with a drop at night to 65°F (18°C) for temperate reptiles and 70°F (21°C) for tropical reptiles, are perfect for most reptiles. The disadvantage of space heaters is that they provide little horizontal thermal gradient. Additional spot heat should be provided by one or more of the following means.

Heat tape and heating pads—A wide variety of these products are now produced specifically for reptiles, especially snakes. Most are capable of burning reptiles if they are in direct contact, even through glass. Heat tape or pads should be placed underneath and at one end of the cage without the full cage weight compressing the pad. Both are capable of melting plastic cages. Heating pads are better for individual cages than heat tape and should be set on low. Heat tape can be run in a strip under one end of a row of cages or coiled under one cage. Flexwatt® heat tape or pads (Flexwatt Corp., 611 Neponset Street, Canton, MA, 02021) are available from most reptile stores or supply catalogs in thin 3- or 11-inch widths that can be cut to the desired length. A rheostat (dimmer switch) can be attached for temperature fine tuning. Rheostats can also control the heat output of most heat sources. Pig blankets, fiberglass-encased resistor pads borrowed from the swine industry, are often used outdoors for spot heat. Keep in mind that species that burrow to escape hot surface temperatures, such as sand boas, *Eryx* sp., or mastigures, *Uromastyx* sp., may burn themselves if heat is provided from below. Perhaps this is because their natural heat avoidance behavior brings them into greater contact with the heat source. Overhead heat is safer for these species.

Incandescent and infrared light bulbs—Lights can be placed above the cage to heat one section of the cage and are especially appropriate for reptiles that bask in the sun regularly (heliotherms). Lights should never be inside the cage without adequate safeguards. Snakes and lizards can lie directly on or under bulbs and severely burn themselves (see figure 1). Lights mounted in the center of the ceiling, well away from the sides, make it more difficult for reptiles to burn themselves. Red or blue lights, or infrared ceramics or lights, should be used at night because continuous light exposure can be stressful to reptiles. Incandescents are available in a wide range of wattages and can be tailored to many different cages. Weatherproof bulbs, or ceramic infrared bulbs, are useful in cages that need to be misted. Infrared bulbs are long lasting, provide a great deal of heat (which is better for larger cages), and are available in a variety of wattages in both glass and ceramic. Keep in mind that infrareds, even ceramic infrareds that produce no visible light, must be mounted far enough from the basking reptile to prevent thermal burns. For instance, with a 250-watt infrared bulb, anything resting within the 18-inch focal plane will eventually burn.

Hot rocks, sizzle stones—These generally do not work well except for some basking lizards and to a lesser extent snakes. They work by directly transferring heat from the heated rock to the reptile and do not typically warm the air. Often the owner comments that the snake or lizard spends all its time on the hot rock, which indicates that the air temperature is too cold. They do not work at all for turtles, as the turtle's shell impairs conductive heat transfer. They are not useful for arboreal reptiles which do not spend time on the floor of the cage. Hot rocks can spontaneously develop local hot spots that may cause burns. Have owners check them periodically for localized hot spots and discard the hot rock if hot spots are present. To prevent burns, the reptile should not come into direct contact with the hot rock.

Be aware that any or all of these heat sources can be a fire hazard. Be sure to observe all electrical codes and avoid overloading outlets. Follow instructions that accompany products, alterations are made at the consumer's own risk.

Humidity

Frye[12] recommends a relative humidity of 50% for xeric (desert) species, 60% to 75% for temperate species, and 80% to 90% for tropical species and amphibians. Neonatal reptiles require higher relative humidity than conspecific adults. Many parts of the country are humid enough that additional humidity is not required. Most desert species do not require increased humidity. Tropical reptiles maintained in drier climates may require a humidifier, especially if electric or forced-air heaters are in use. Humidity can be boosted by covering cage openings with clear plastic, increasing the surface area of water bowls, providing a hide box with damp vermiculite or sphagnum moss, or placing a damp sponge under a hide box. Directing heat at the water bowl and occasional misting of the cage with a handheld sprayer will increase relative humidity. Live plants also boost humidity. When very high humidity is needed, an aquarium heater in a water-filled container can be placed in the cage.[55] Low humidity predisposes reptiles to difficulty in shedding, respiratory disease and dehydration. Humidifiers can support bacterial and fungal growth. This can be a potential health hazard if water is nebulized throughout the air. Good air circulation is important, and humidifiers should be disinfected regularly. Ultrasonic humidifiers support much less bacterial and fungal growth than steam humidifiers.

Cage Accessories

Newspaper is recommended for hospital use because it is cheap, easily noticed when soiled or wet, and easy to clean. Most reptiles benefit from a hide box. A hide box is a small container that the reptile can crawl into or under and get out of sight. Some reptiles, especially snakes, are positively thigmotropic, which means that they orient to maximize the stimulus of touch or contact. Hide boxes are believed to reduce stress in reptiles by making them feel more secure in their enclosure. They should be just large enough that the reptile fits in with little extra space. Hide boxes can be made out of many materials, but plastic commercial reptile hide boxes are easiest to clean and disinfect in the hospital. Arboreal lizards and snakes prefer raised hide boxes. Visual barriers such as heavy foliage are important for tropical arboreal lizards, as are branches. Hardwood driftwood branches cut to the size of the cage work well, or branches can be purchased from pet stores. Branches should be scrubbed with hot water and need to be kept clean. For arboreal snakes, polyvinyl chloride (PVC) tubing works well. Artificial silk leaves or plants are not recommended because of their potential for being eaten or causing toxicity (from water soluble stiffeners sprayed on them during manufacture) and because some lizards are unable to climb on them.[56]

Water bowls should be present for all reptiles. Make sure they are drinking from the bowl! If they will not drink from a bowl, administer water with a syringe, mist their cage, or soak them in shallow (¼ to ½ inch), lukewarm (80°F [27°C]) water. Be careful when soaking reptiles because they can drown easily if the water is too deep. Certain species (anoles, chameleons, chuckawallas, other small tropical iguanids and agamids, rough green snakes, and ribbon snakes) won't drink well from water bowls and must be misted, or provided with a drip system.

Ultraviolet Lights

An area of considerable debate and uncertainty within the herpetocultural world is the need for ultraviolet (UV) lights. Ultraviolet irradiation in the 290- to 320-nanometer (nm) wavelength is necessary for photochemical activation of cholecalciferol (vitamin D_3) in mammals. It seems reasonable to assume this holds true for reptiles and amphibians as well, especially because they also utilize cholecalciferol. Snakes seem to be the lone exception. Perhaps snakes do not require UV light as a consequence of their fossorial evolution. For all other reptiles, sunlight is the best source of UV light and should be provided whenever feasible. Unfortunately, glass and most plastics filter out UV light; therefore, sunlight passing through glass windows cannot provide UV light for indoor animals. If the window is open, screening still allows UV penetration with only a slight decrease in transmittance. Special UV transmissible glass and plastics are available but costly.

Uncertainty arises when reptiles move indoors away from unfiltered sunlight. For short periods (an educated guess would be less than three or four months) reptiles should be able to utilize stored vitamin D. For longer periods, alternatives are needed to sustain vitamin D metabolism. An alternative to UV light would be to provide preformed vitamin D_3 in the diet. Studies indicate that vitamin D_3 is 10 to 20 times more toxic than vitamin D_2.[57] For most animals the presumed maximum safe level of vitamin D_3 for long-term feeding conditions (more than two months) is 4 to 10 times the recognized dietary requirement.[57] Cholecalciferol supplementation is potentially dangerous because dietary requirements for vitamin D remain unknown for all reptiles. In addition, vitamin D is fat soluble and thus retained in the body even if oversupplemented. In other words, we are considering an unknown dosage of a potentially toxic substance with a narrow spectrum of safety. To confuse the issue further, it is not at all clear that all reptiles utilize oral vitamin D and substantial differences may exist between different species. Be aware that large amounts of vitamin D are present in multivitamins, most reptile calcium supplements, and fortified chows. From the author's perspective, until more is known, it seems prudent to limit multivitamin supplementation (to no more than once or twice a month) and seek other methods for regulating vitamin D. During warmer months, with regular outdoor basking, dietary vitamin D can be curtailed.

A reasonable option indoors is to provide artificial UV lights. Much debate exists over the use of artificial sources of UV light. Broad-spectrum lights, with some UV output between 290 and 320 nm, are hypothesized to stimulate cholecalciferol synthesis in reptiles. Unfortunately, this hypothesis remains unproved despite widespread usage of UV lights for the past several decades. However, empirical evidence does support the use of artificial UV lights. Many experienced herpetoculturists recommend that when reptiles cannot regularly bask outdoors for extended periods, fluorescent UV lights should be provided for approximately 12 hours per day. A timer is recommended to keep the photoperiod regular. Two-bulb fluorescent light fixtures with a black light (Sylvania) and either a Vitalite (Durotest Corp.), Chroma-50 (General Electric), or Colortone 50 (Westinghouse, North American Philips Lighting Corp.) have been used by herpetoculturists for years. Combination of fluorescents is beneficial because black lights produce slightly more UV light (particularly UV A) but little visible light. Combining a black light with other fluorescents produces brighter visible light. Divers[58] mentioned that anorexia in iguanas housed under black lights improved when they were switched to more balanced light. In recent years there has been a surge in UV lights specifically designed for reptiles. It is difficult to evaluate critically the differences between lights but, in general, they have much more UV B spectral output. As UV B light serves as a photochemical catalyst in cholecalciferol activation, the percentage of UV B spectral output may be much less important than the simple presence or absence of the right wavelength. As UV light intensity decreases exponentially with increasing distance, the lights should be within 24 inches of the reptile, many recommend 12 to 18 inches. Replace UV lights every 18 months, or sooner, as ultraviolet output decreases precipitously after this age. Plant lights and incandescent lights do not produce UV B light.

Sunlamps are an alternative form of UV light but in a much more concentrated form. Sunlamps are restricted to use in the medical community and are not available to the general public. They can burn reptiles (as well as humans) with heat and UV light and their use should be discouraged. In some zoos they are used in very large enclosures where they are kept a minimum of 6 feet from the animal. Fluorescent lights are much safer for smaller enclosures. Further studies on basking reptiles are desperately needed to determine whether UV lights are effective in activation of vitamin D.

Incubation of Reptile Eggs

The most widely used incubation medium is vermiculite (heat-expanded mica), available from most commercial nurseries, garden supply stores, or plant sections of some grocery stores. Coarse grade no. 3 vermiculite is preferable to finer vermiculite.[59] Vermiculite is mixed with water in an equal ratio by weight, such as one part vermiculite to one part water.[60] In other words, if one uses 200 grams of vermiculite, 200 ml of water should be added. Some breeders feel that a more arid substrate (such as 1 part vermiculite to 0.4 part water) may improve hatching success in colubrids.[61] The vermiculite and water should be mixed well and placed in a clean plastic shoe box, gallon jar, or some other sealable container large enough to contain the eggs. Some breeders like to leave a small open water container (such as a film canister) in with the eggs to further boost humidity for humid species.[62] Eggs are transferred gently with clean hands to the incubation chamber in the orientation in which they were laid. Do not try to separate clumped eggs. Eggs should be buried halfway in the incubation medium and the container briefly opened every several days to facilitate respiration. Other incubation media that work well for many people include perlite, peat moss, sphagnum moss, sand, and paper towels. The author prefers vermiculite because of extensive experience with it. Perlite is less hydroscopic than vermiculite, which keeps water down at the bottom of the container and away from the eggs but still maintains humidity. Many reptile breeders are convinced that this makes a difference. Given the proper oxygen, humidity, and temperature requirements, reptile eggs can hatch with almost any incubation medium.

Incubate temperate and tropical species at 27 to 29°C (80 to 85°F) until hatching. Python eggs should be incubated at 30 to 32°C (86 to 90°F). Certain species, such as chameleons and some geckos, are often incubated at lower temperatures. An incubator is essential if room temperatures are not stable or warm enough. A simple incubator can be made from a polystyrene (Styrofoam) box raised above a heating pad until the desired temperature is achieved. A submersible aquarium heater in an aquarium partially filled with water can provide thermostatically stable heat for an egg container resting on the water's surface. A variety of other incubators can be purchased or fabricated. The author uses a simple plywood box heated with an 11-inch-wide Flexwatt heating pad and a thermostat. Stable egg temperatures are crucial to hatching success. Setting up the incubator with the egg container several days prior to egg production is important to allow temperatures to equalize. An accurate minimum–maximum thermometer is crucial (see temperature section in this chapter).

Length of incubation is temperature and species dependent. Higher temperatures usually decrease the incubation time up to a certain limit. Fiber-optic candling devices are excellent for checking fertility. Fertile squamate (snake and lizard) eggs remain creamy white or sometimes pinkish, slowly swell with incubation, and develop minute blood vessels visible by candling. Also with candling, fertile chelonian eggs develop a small opaque area dorsally that gradually spreads ventrally (the so-called chalk line; see figure 2). Infertile or dead eggs often grow mold, desiccate, collapse, discolor, or are dull yellowish white. If the eggs look good and start dimpling, they could be drying out, unless near hatching. Evaporative water loss desiccates substrates and eggs; a little misting of the substrate or water addition should allow the eggs to fill back out. If the entire egg container is weighed at the start of incubation, the weight loss in grams over time equals the evaporative water loss in milliliters, which can then be periodically accurately replenished. If eggs continue to dimple with humid conditions, they are probably no longer fertile or never were. If the eggs swell so much that they develop translucent streaks, the medium is too wet. Raising them above the incubation medium and removing the water container, if present, will allow them to dry partially.[59,62] One can visually check the eggs, but remember that picking up or rolling eggs can be very hard on developing embryos.

It is best to allow hatchlings to emerge from the egg on their own, which can take several hours to several days. Until the yolk sac is resorbed (usually within several days; see figures 3 to 5), it is best to house them on clean, damp paper towels or let them remain in the egg container. Squamates typically hatch within several days of one another. If most of the clutch has hatched, the remaining eggs can be carefully slit with iris scissors.

Crocodilians, most turtles, and many lizards have temperature-dependent sex determination, whereas snakes and some lizards have genetic sex determination (sex chromosomes). Complicating temperature-dependent sex-determination research is the discovery that only during certain critical periods of incubation does temperature affect the sex that will be produced.

Salmonella

Reptiles are well-known reservoirs for a variety of unusual *Salmonella* serotypes. The rarity of some of these serotypes often allows epidemiologists to trace human infections back to reptiles. In 1972 the Centers for Disease Control and Prevention banned the importation of turtles less than 4 inches in length, and in 1975 the Food and Drug Administration prohibited the interstate transport of the turtles to thwart an epidemic of turtle-associated salmonellosis in children. Children were unable to cram turtles over 4 inches in length into their mouths, so larger turtles were deemed less of a risk. What many do not realize is that *Salmonella* is just as common, if not more common, in snakes, lizards, and crocodilians. Indeed most, if not all, reptiles are thought to carry *Salmonella*.[63] *Salmonella* can survive in cages for as long as 6 months after the reptile was present[64] and in avian or bovine feces for as long as 28 to 30 months.[65] *Salmonella* is easily spread through bathtubs, clothing, hands, or carpets, which provides further incentive not to turn reptiles loose in one's house. Salmonellosis in infants has frequently been traced back to reptiles and is particularly dangerous. In many instances the infant had no direct contact with the reptile. *Salmonella* exposure in most people causes few to no symptoms. However, in certain people it can be much more serious, with symptoms ranging from abdominal cramps, profuse bloody diarrhea, fever, headache, and lack of appetite to vomiting, muscle pain, sepsis, and death.

All reptiles should be considered potential asymptomatic carriers of *Salmonella.* Asymptomatic carriage rates for iguanas in California have been found to be 60% to 80%.[66] Negative fecal culture, even if performed on several consecutive fecal samples, does not mean the reptile is free from *Salmonella*. *Salmonella* may be shed intermittently or under periods of stress. Repeated studies have shown that treatment of healthy lizards and turtles for *Salmonella*, with appropriate antibiotics, does not eliminate *Salmonella* and may actually prolong shedding.[66–68] For instance, iguanas treated for *Salmonella* reverted to a culture-positive state within 3 to 5 months after treatment.[66] Furthermore, treatment may increase antibiotic resistance. Given these facts, routine screening of reptiles for *Salmonella* is not recommended. Rather, assume that *Salmonella* is present in reptiles and observe the following recommendations for prevention of its transmission from reptiles to humans offered by the Centers for Disease Control and Prevention[69] (with some additional comments).

1. Persons at increased risk for infection or serious complications of salmonellosis (e.g., pregnant women, children younger than 5 years old, and immunocompromised per-

sons, such as persons with acquired immunodeficiency syndrome [AIDS]) should avoid contact with reptiles and their cages.

2. Reptiles should not be kept in child care centers and may not be appropriate pets in households in which persons at increased risk for infection reside.

3. Veterinary hospitals and pet stores should provide information to owners and potential purchasers of reptiles about the increased risk of acquiring *Salmonella* from reptiles.

4. Veterinary and pet store workers should advise reptile owners always to wash their hands with warm soapy water (antibacterial soaps are preferred) after handling reptiles or reptile cages and not to eat or put anything in their mouth while working with reptiles. Allowing free roaming of the house by reptiles and kissing reptiles should be discouraged.

5. To prevent contamination of food preparation areas (e.g., kitchens) and other selected sites, reptiles should be kept out of these areas. In particular, kitchens or infant bathing areas should not be used to bathe reptiles or to wash reptile dishes or cages. Discard soiled material into a toilet or trash can. Clean water bowls in a sink not used for bathing or drinking or thoroughly clean such areas afterward.

Keep in mind that one is much more likely to be exposed to *Salmonella* from raw or inadequately cooked poultry or eggs. Most people who are exposed to *Salmonella* do not develop illness. With a little common sense and good hygiene, salmonellosis is easily avoided. If veterinarians are called upon to assist health officials in a human *Salmonella* case, combined fecal and cloacal cultures from reptiles are recommended.

Quarantine of Reptiles

Quarantine of all new additions to larger collections for 3 to 6 (snakes) months is strongly recommended.[70,71] Three months is generally longer than past recommendations. This interval gives the keeper adequate time to detect and treat for parasites and be certain the reptile is healthy and eating well. The major objectives of quarantine are to prevent introduction of serious reptilian diseases such as amebiasis, cryptosporidiosis, inclusion body disease of boids, mites, ophidian paramyxovirus infection, and upper respiratory tract disease in chelonians.[70] Other parasites are a lesser concern but should still be treated.

As early in quarantine as practical, reptiles should be weighed and have a complete physical and fecal examination. Fecal examination should include fecal flotations (for detection of trematodes, nematodes, cestodes, protozoans, and pentastomids), fresh direct fecal smears (for easier detection of certain protozoans), and, if affordable, acid-fast stains (for detection of cryptosporidia or acid-fast bacteria). For valuable animals, blood work may be indicated to evaluate health further. Any animals that are not eating well, losing weight, or diseased should not be released from quarantine. Consider euthanasia and necropsy of animals that chronically do not do well and any animal that dies during quarantine. Repeated fecal examinations after treatment are advisable to ensure anthelmintic effectiveness.

Multiple quarantine facilities are desirable, several for incoming animals and at least one for sick animals. Sick and incoming quarantined animals should never be mixed. If multiple facilities are available, all in and all out quarantine is possible. Quarantine facilities should be isolated as much as possible from the main facility. Ideally, separate facilities are indicated. Minimally, separate ventilation systems and sinks are indicated. The quarantine facility should be serviced last after the main facility. There should be no exchange of anything from quarantine to the main collection. This includes cages, snake hooks, food items, and cleaning utensils. Wear gloves and, if possible, separate clothes or gowns in the quarantine facility to further limit spread of pathogens. Shipping material from other facilities should be opened in quarantine and then promptly thrown out.

Most zoos and serious breeders are beginning to appreciate the importance of quarantine. The aforementioned serious diseases occur frequently enough that they will eventually infect larger collections that are not properly quarantined. When one considers the expense of lost animals and veterinary work-up and the difficulty in establishing which animals were exposed to or are carriers of a major pathogen, quarantine becomes a much more cost-effective alternative. For breeders, quarantine is a basic measure to protect their livelihood. A limited quarantine period is better than none. The intensity of quarantine ultimately depends on the keeper and how valuable the collection is. As with anything in veterinary medicine, explain the options and let clients choose the level of care they are comfortable with.

2

Turtles, Tortoises, and Terrapins*

General Considerations

Taxonomy

Turtles, tortoises, and terrapins are collectively referred to as chelonians because they are all members of the order Chelonia (also referred to as Testudines, Testudinata). The common names of chelonians vary throughout the world and change from language to language.[72] Tortoise usually refers to terrestrial turtles, such as members of the family Testudinidae. Australians, however, refer to all but one of their turtles as tortoises, despite the fact that no true tortoises exist there and all of their chelonians are aquatic. In the United Kingdom, terrapin refers to freshwater chelonians, turtle refers to marine chelonians, and tortoise refers to terrestrial chelonians. In North America, turtle refers to both aquatic and terrestrial chelonians and terrapins can be freshwater or marine. One can begin to appreciate the value of scientific names that are the same from language to language.

There are two suborders of chelonians, the Cryptodirans (hidden-neck turtles) and the Pleurodirans (side-neck turtles). There are a number of anatomical differences between these groups, the most recognizable of which is the mode of head retraction. Cryptodiran turtles are able to retract their necks straight back into their shells, thereby hiding both head and neck. Pleurodirans are not able to retract the neck; instead they fold it up sideways, hence their common name side-necks or snake-necks. Unfortunately for veterinarians, cryptodirans provide the majority of turtles commonly seen. Veterinarians who have struggled to get a cryptodiran turtle's head out of its shell may not realize what a cruel twist of fate evolution has produced for us.

*This chapter was revised, with permission, from Boyer and Boyer.[76]

Captive care of chelonians is a challenge because the 240 or more species have evolved to thrive in many different habitats. In general, chelonians require much more space than lizards or snakes. The majority of turtles seen in private practice are box turtles, tortoises, and aquatic turtles. Therefore this chapter will focus on some general considerations about these turtles and their specific care. Remember that for such a diverse group a summary of captive care is overly simplified. Good information on natural history and captive care is essential (see Highfield[73] for more information).

Predators

Predators, especially dogs, are fond of chewing on chelonian shells and appendages and can wreak havoc in a very short time (see figure 6). Small chelonians can be devoured without a trace. Raccoons and opossums enter yards at night to prey on turtles. Other mammals and birds are also potential predators. Smaller terrestrial and all aquatic chelonians should always have screened outdoor cages.

Hibernation

Hibernation is recommended for temperate species, such as northernly distributed box turtles (*Terrapene carolina carolina*, *Terrapene c. triunguis*, *Terrapene ornata ornata*), several tortoise species (*Testudo marginata*, *T. hermanni*, most *T. graeca*, *T. horsfieldi*, and *Gopherus agassizii*, *G. polyphemus*, and *G. berlandieri*), and many aquatic turtles. *Terrapene bauri* and *Terrapene c. major* do not hibernate. Keep in mind that within a given species animals from warmer areas or econiches may not hibernate at all. Some temperate species may skip hibernation in captivity, especially if the conditions stay warm and the day remains artificially long. Others, particularly box turtles, stop eating in the early fall regardless of artificial conditions. Hibernation is recommended for healthy specimens of good body weight.

In order to survive hibernation, the turtle must have good body weight and good health. A physical examination several weeks prior to hibernation is advisable. Sick, convalescing, or underweight turtles (evidenced by swollen eyelids, sunken eyes, nasal discharge, laborious or gurgling respiration) should not be hibernated! Weight gain over the summer is a prerequisite for hibernation. Jackson's ratio compares body weight to carapace length and is a simple and accurate method of assessing tortoise health (see weight evaluation in the section Basic Medical Techniques for Turtles, Tortoises, and Terrapins later in this chapter).

Most chelonians that hibernate will noticeably decrease their food intake as hibernation approaches. Water should be constantly available prior to hibernation; soaking encourages drinking. In early October, or as soon as the turtle's appetite noticeably decreases in early fall, withhold food (but not water) for 1 to 2 weeks for smaller turtles and up to 3 weeks for larger tortoises, but keep the turtle between 21 and 27°C (70 and 80°F). This gives the turtle time to clear its gastrointestinal tract of potentially fermentable ingesta. After this, remove external heat sources and allow the turtle to acclimate to a room temperature of 16 to 21°C (60 to 70°F). After a week at room temperature, the turtle should be ready to enter the hibernaculum.

Chelonians can be hibernated indoors or outdoors. Outdoor hibernation is potentially more dangerous, because one has less control over environmental conditions. For indoor hibernation, select an area that can be kept between 2 and 10°C (35 and 50°F) for the winter, such as a basement, garage, back porch, crawl space, wine cellar, or north- or east-facing closet, window, or wall. Use a minimum–maximum thermometer to check temperatures several weeks before hibernation. Persistent temperatures above 16°C (60°F) are not cool enough for hibernation, and the turtle's metabolism will be high enough that it will slowly starve. Prolonged temperatures below 2°C (35°F) are too cold; temperatures below freezing should be avoided.

A hibernaculum can be set up with a large box, crate, cooler, or aquarium with a foot of slightly humid peat-based potting soil and a 3- to

6-inch layer of shredded newspaper, dried leaves, or hay on top. Make sure the hibernarium is not resting directly on cold cement. The turtle should burrow into the soil and remain inactive. The soil should be humid enough that the turtle does not dehydrate but should not be wet.

If low humidity is a problem indoors, consider periodic soaking to prevent dehydration. Chelonians can be awakened every 2 to 4 weeks and allowed to drink or soak in shallow 24°C (75°F) water for 2 hours.[74] During soaking, the turtle's eyes should reopen. If the turtle appears healthy, let it dry off and then return it to the hibernaculum. If any signs of illness are present warm the turtle up to 27°C (80°F) and begin antibiotic treatment immediately. Contrary to popular belief, disturbing turtles during hibernation is not harmful.[73]

Species that naturally hibernate in a given geographic area can be hibernated outdoors. Outdoor hibernation is not advisable in areas with severe winters. For box turtles select an area sheltered from the wind with 2 to 3 feet of loosened soil; loose soil near a foundation works well. Spread a foot or two of loose leaves or hay over the soil. The turtle will burrow into the soil and attempt to stay below the frost line. Be sure the area drains well and is not prone to flooding. Compost areas are not good for hibernation.

Tortoises can be hibernated outdoors in milder climates in artificial burrows or doghouses. A burrow can be constructed with partially or fully buried concrete blocks along the sides and ¾-inch plywood on the top. Leave a southern exposure entrance covered with a heavy tarp or opaque plastic and place hay or straw inside. A simpler alternative is a well-insulated doghouse filled with a thick layer of leaves or soil. Place a tarp or plastic over the entrance. Outdoor hibernacula should be protected against freezing and flooding. Low humidity is generally not a problem outdoors, but turtles should still be encouraged to drink if active on warmer days.

Typically, chelonians hibernate outdoors for five to six months from mid-October until early April. Indoor hibernation can be shorter, from early November to late February or early March. Highfield[73] recommends 8 to 10 weeks for small specimens and no longer than 12 to 14 weeks for large specimens. Once the turtle becomes active in the spring, it should be soaked in lukewarm water and start eating well within a week or two. Healthy tortoises should lose less than 6% to 7% of their body weight over the winter hibernation.[74]

Hibernation of juveniles is controversial.[73] Some feel turtles less than 3 to 4 years of age should not hibernate. Much depends on the experience of the keeper and the stability of hibernaculum temperatures. When in doubt, it does not hurt to skip hibernation for the first few years.

Box Turtle Care

Introduction

Box turtles are one of the most common reptile pets in the United States. With proper care they are long-lived, with life spans of 30 to 40 years and perhaps much longer. Unfortunately, they are among the most neglected reptiles in captivity, because most people do not appreciate how to care for them properly.

Taxonomy

Several subspecies of box turtle are common in the pet trade, including the eastern box turtle (*Terrapene carolina carolina*), Gulf Coast box turtle (*Terrapene c. major*), Florida box turtle (*Terrapene c. bauri*), three-toed box turtle (*Terrapene c. triungius*), ornate box turtle (*Terrapene ornata ornata*), and desert box turtle (*Terrapene o. luteola*).

Reproduction

Most species lay two to eight (normally four to six) eggs from May through July. Multiple clutches are possible. Females can store sperm and lay fertile eggs for up to 4 years after fertilization. Eggs hatch in 2 to 3 months if fertile (see incubation section in chapter 1).

Housing

Twenty-gallon aquariums are the minimum size for box turtles. Consider larger aquariums or make larger cages out of plywood (see tortoise care later in this chapter) or use concrete mixing containers available in most hardware stores. The bigger the enclosure, the better. The bottom of the cage should be filled with a humid substrate such as medium to large wood chips mixed with peat moss or a sand and soil mixture. Drier substrates promote skin cracking and poor health. Substrates need to be changed completely every few months and feces need to be scooped out on a weekly basis. A hide box that the turtle can get under and out of sight is important. Many turtles prefer to sleep in them. Loose leaf litter can be spread in the cage.

Temperature

The indoor cage should get no colder than 15°C (60°F) at night and gradually warm to 21 to 27°C (70 to 80°F) during the day. A 75- to 100-watt incandescent bulb with reflector can provide a warm basking area at one end of the cage between 27 and 32°C (80 and 90°F). Lights should be turned off during the night, so supplemental heat from heat tape or heating pads also should be provided under one-half of the cage if temperatures drop below 15°C (60°F). Hot rocks do not work well for turtles.

Outdoor housing

During the late spring, summer, and early fall months, turtles do best outdoors in a backyard or fenced enclosure. Provide shade with dense shrubbery, dry leaves, or a wooden shelter so that turtles can escape the hot sun when needed. Box turtles are good at digging under fences and escaping. Often this explains the observation of so many proud, new box-turtle owners that "it just wandered into our yard." The yard perimeter should be carefully sealed with bricks, rocks, boards, or buried fencing and periodically patrolled for developing breaks. Box turtles can also climb over fencing less than 12 inches high.[75] Bring turtles indoors whenever the temperature drops into the low 60s (15 to 18°C).

Water

An easy-to-clean, shallow water dish, big enough for the turtle to get into, should always be available. Water should be no deeper than the turtle's chin when its head is partially retracted. Turtles prefer to defecate in their water bowl, so it should be cleaned several times per week. Juvenile box turtles are often much more aquatic than adults. Box turtles drown in deep water, such as in a swimming pool. Highfield[73] notes that *Terrapene c. bauri* and *Terrapene c. triunguis* are better swimmers than other box turtles and even forage under water.

Feeding

Box turtles are much more carnivorous than most people realize. Adult eastern box turtles are opportunistic omnivores consuming land snails, beetles, sowbugs or pillbugs, millipedes, slugs, earthworms, spiders, carrion, small mammals, birds, crayfish, frogs, tadpoles, salamanders, lizards, snakes, smaller turtles, and plant material such as mushrooms, strawberries, raspberries, mulberries, and tomatoes. Youngsters are primarily carnivorous. Ornate box turtles are mainly insectivorous, consuming dung beetles, caterpillars, cicadas, and grasshoppers, but they also eat mulberries, leaves, tender shoots, and carrion. Unlike other box turtles, ornates frequently utilize burrows and prefer a more arid habitat such as open prairie.

In captivity, chronic nutritional problems are typical for most box turtles yet difficult to appreciate. Nutritional diseases can be avoided by feeding a well-balanced diet that is continually varied. The following is one recommended diet;[76] items listed in bold print are box turtle favorites and often entice finicky turtles to eat. Keep in mind that different species have different dietary preferences. For instance, ornates are much more carnivorous and thus less interested in plant material. Ornates often thrive on a mixed diet of insects and mice. Interpret these guidelines liberally.

50% Animal or High-protein Foods—Examples include: **earthworms; crickets; grasshoppers; cicadas; slugs; snails; whole-skinned chopped mice; baby mice (pinkies)**; waxworms; mealworms; super mealworms; silk moth larvae; other insects; adult, low-fat maintenance dog chow; trout; parrot or turtle chows; and goldfish. The vitamin-fortified chows should be limited to **less than 5%** of the total diet because of the high vitamin, fat, and protein content. All dry chows should be soaked in water for 30 minutes to soften them. Avoid cat food because it is too high in fat and protein for reptiles. Do not add multivitamins to foods that are already vitamin fortified. Feed a wide variety of animal and high-protein foods, not just a few of these items. Insects are calcium deficient and should be fed enriched diets dusted with powdered calcium carbonate, lactate, citrate, or gluconate just before offering them to the turtle (see feeding insectivorous reptiles and amphibians in chapter 4).

50% Plants: 25% Fruits and 75% Vegetables—

25% Fruits—Fruits are tasty but mineral deficient, so they must be limited. Turtles are fond of **tomatoes, strawberries, raspberries,** apples, grapes, cherries, peaches, pears, plums, oranges, nectarines, figs, melons (remove seeds), bananas, mangoes, and grapefruit.

> *75% Vegetables*—Varied vegetables include dark leafy greens (mustard, collard, radish, beet and turnip greens or tops); kale; cabbage; spinach; red leaf or romaine lettuce; **dandelions (leaves, stems, and flowers)**; bok choy; pak choi; broccoli rabe; squashes; sweet potatoes; carrots; thawed frozen mixed vegetables (peas, corn, carrots, green beans, and lima beans); carrots (shaved, not chopped); alfalfa; radish; clover or bean sprouts; **mushrooms**; red, green, or yellow bell peppers; broccoli; green beans; peas in the pod; okra; and prickly pear cactus pads (shave off spines). Wash fruits and vegetables and chop all items into bite-sized pieces. Some species, such as ornate and Gulf Coast box turtles, are not fond of vegetables. Mixing vegetables well with other foods will often encourage consumption.

Box turtles have a continuous need for foods rich in vitamin A. Liver (in whole mice) is an excellent source of vitamin A, as well as rich yellow or dark orange vegetables (carrots, sweet potatoes, butternut and winter squashes) and dark leafy greens (dandelion greens and flowers, spinach, turnip, and mustard greens). Steaming (not boiling) hard squashes makes them much more palatable and easier to chop.

Adults should be fed three or more times per week in the morning and juveniles daily. Every feeding to every other feeding, lightly dust food with calcium lactate, carbonate, citrate, or gluconate. Every 2 to 4 weeks, dust food lightly with multivitamins if vitamin-fortified foods are not eaten. Oversupplementation with multivitamins is not healthy. Feed as much variety as possible to ensure a healthy balanced diet!

For finicky eaters, try some of their favorite foods (listed in bold print) and keep in mind that box turtles are particularly attracted to red-, yellow-, and orange-colored foods. Live, moving food will often stimulate feeding; pinkies and earthworms often entice the most recalcitrant specimens to feed. Box turtles are most active in early morning or late afternoon, when it is not too hot, so these are good times to try to feed them. Rainstorms often increase activity; thus, spraying their cage can stimulate appetite. When you find something they really like, mix it heavily into the salad and then gradually decrease it over a period of weeks. Bad dietary habits can be difficult to overcome and often require months to correct. Continue to offer foods even if they are not eaten initially, as the turtle adjusts to a varied salad, it will gradually increase dietary diversity.

Acclimatization

Most pet box turtles are wild-caught adults and may adapt poorly to captivity, although some do well from the start. If healthy, new arrivals should be set up in as large a cage as possible or placed outdoors if the weather is favorable. They are naturally secretive animals, and frequent handling or watching will deter them from settling into captivity.

Tortoise Care

Taxonomy

The true tortoises are all members of the family Testudinidae, which encompasses 12 genera with 40 living species. Common temperate species include desert tortoises (*Gopherus agassizii*), gopher tortoises (*G. polyphemus*), Hermann's tortoise (*Testudo hermanni*), Russian tortoises (*T. horsfieldi*), and Greek tortoises (*T. graeca*). Common tropical species include red-footed tortoises (*Geochelone carbonaria*), yellow-footed tortoises (*G. denticulata*), spurred tortoises (*G. sulcata*), leopard tortoises (*G. pardalis*), and hinged, or hinge-backed, tortoises (*Kinixys* spp.).

Outdoor housing

Whenever possible, tortoises should be kept outdoors, even if only for a small portion of the year. This allows them space to exercise, graze, and bask in the sun, which is important for vitamin D synthesis. Well-acclimated, adult tropical tortoises can be housed outdoors when morning temperatures are above 18°C (65°F) and midday temperatures exceed 24°C (75°F). Bring them in at night when temperatures are below 18°C (65°F) or provide a heated outdoor enclosure. Adult temperate species tolerate temperatures 3°C (5°F) less than those listed for tropical species. For small juveniles, temperatures should always be above 24°C (75°F) (see neonatal care later in this chapter).

Tethering a tortoise by a leg or through a hole in the shell is not acceptable and is potentially harmful. Leg tethers can cut into flesh and result in severe infection. Drilling a hole through the shell should be considered inhumane.

When planning outdoor enclosures, several factors should be considered. Desert species can tolerate higher temperatures and drier enclosures than tropical rainforest species. Outdoor enclosures can be modified to suit the needs of species. For tropical forest forms, such as *Geochelone carbonaria*, *G. denticulata*, *Manouria emys*, *Kinixys homeana*, *K. erosa*, *K. belliana*, and *Indotestudo* spp., densely planted enclosures are ideal. For grassland, or desert species, such as *Gopherus* and *Testudo* spp., *Geochelone sulcata*, and *G. pardalis*, enclosures can be more sparsely planted with shrubs and grasses. In either type of enclosure, shelters should be provided for retreat from the elements as well as shade.

Outdoor enclosures should have secure perimeters. Tortoises generally pace at the perimeters and constantly try to get through perimeters they can see through. Therefore, solid barriers, such as wooden fencing or smooth concrete, at tortoise eye level is preferable to open fencing. Chicken wire can entrap and cut tortoise legs and is not advisable. Ideally, one should bury 6 to 12 inches of perimeter fencing to prevent underground escape.

Outdoor hazards

In the southeastern United States fire ants (*Solenopis* spp.) can attack and kill small tortoises. Another potential threat, especially in residential areas, is pesticide spraying. Do not spray tortoise enclosures with pesticides. Instruct owners to have their neighbors inform them when they apply pesticides so that their tortoises can be removed to a safer area.

Tortoises will consume all the vegetation growing in their enclosure. Therefore, toxic plants should be removed (see Frye[16] for a list of toxic plants). Most grasses, clover, perennial legumes, and dandelions are suitable. Tortoises will also eat a variety of nonfood items in their cage. Enclosures should be regularly examined for scraps of metal, nails, wire, pieces of plastic, and other trash that blows in. Tortoises also consume small rocks and pebbles; generally, these are no cause for concern. For more information, see the section on predators earlier in this chapter.

Indoor housing

Indoor housing is usually mandatory for a good portion of the year, except in subtropical areas. Tortoises require more space than most reptiles. The New York Turtle and Tortoise Society recommends that the combined shell size of all tortoises present should not exceed a quarter of the floor surface area available to the tortoises.[77]

Aquariums, plastic or metal livestock troughs, concrete mixing containers, or plastic sweater boxes can be used for small tortoises. Cages can be constructed for larger tortoises with ½- to ¾-inch plywood on the bottom and two 2 by 12 inch planks stacked on one another or plywood along the sides. The inner cage surfaces should be caulked and sealed with an undercoat of water sealant and two to three coats of polyurethane, or one can use melamine. Sealing exposed wood surfaces facilitates cleaning and disinfecting. Allow the cage to air out thoroughly (usually about a week) before placing any tortoises in it.

To prevent chilling, the cage bottom should not be in direct contact with cold concrete; a gap of 4 to 6 inches is advisable. An alternative to building a cage is to convert a garage or unfinished room into a tortoise pen.

Ambient indoor temperature should be 24 to 32°C (75 to 90°F), depending on the species. Rooms can be heated with thermostatically controlled space heaters. A thermogradiant should be provided with basking lights and/or heating pads (see temperature section in chapter 1).

Substrates

Juveniles are often maintained on alfalfa pellets and, as they graduate to larger cages, a mixture of medium to large conifer bark nuggets and peat moss. Acceptable alternative substrates include newspaper, indoor–outdoor carpeting (be sure to avoid frayed edges), or corrugated cardboard. Remove fecal material from the enclosure several times per week and replace the substrate several times per year. For very large enclosures and large species, smooth cement, clean soil (baseball infield soil or soil with a high clay content), or hay can be used, provided the room stays warm. Avoid sand, gravel, clay cat litter, and crushed corncob or walnut shells. Many tortoises are reclusive animals. As with outdoor enclosures, a shelter or hidebox should be provided.

Water

Water should be regularly available for indoor and outdoor tortoises. Shallow plastic plant saucers work well for small tortoises. Make sure the water is no more than chin deep or the tortoise may accidentally overturn and drown. Larger plastic containers or cooking pans work well for medium-sized tortoises. For large tortoises, one can notch the side of a plastic shoe box or sink pan, and tortoises will use it.

Tortoises often defecate in their water; thus, water bowls should be changed daily, every other day, or whenever dirty. Tortoises outdoors will also drink from standing water.

An alternative to water bowls is to soak the tortoises in chin-deep water three times per week. This option is less desirable in that invariably one occasionally forgets to soak tortoises. The resulting intermittent dehydration may contribute to formation of uroliths and gout.

Feeding

Diets for captive tortoises are an area of considerate-owner uncertainty and variability. Wild tortoises often utilize forage of a relatively low nutritional value. In captivity, diets tend to have a much higher nutritional value, which may not be beneficial in the long run. Empirically, the author has had success with a diet that includes 95% vegetables, less than 5% fruit, and very small amounts of high-protein foods, or none of the latter.

> **95% Vegetables**—The majority of vegetables should be dark leafy greens (mustard, collard, radish, and turnip greens or tops, kale, cabbage, dandelions [leaves, stems, and flowers], bok choy, pak choi, broccoli rabe and backyard grasses, clovers, legumes, and weeds (freshly cut or as browse). Feed less spinach, Swiss chard, beet greens, and red leaf or romaine lettuce. Mulberry, hibiscus and grape leaves, roses, nasturtiums, hibiscus, carnation, and squash flowers are good, as are soaked alfalfa pellets, thawed frozen mixed vegetables (peas, corn, carrots, green and lima beans), peas in the pod, cauliflower, green beans, alfalfa, clover, radish or soy bean sprouts, jicama, green peppers, radishes, summer and winter squashes, and prickly pear cactus pads (shave off spines).
>
> Cured alfalfa, timothy, or Bermuda grass works well for large tortoises if one can get them used to eating it. Soaking hay in water for an hour prior to offering it may

increase palatability, especially if it is mixed with salad. Fresh green grasses are always preferable. Green, uncured alfalfa is a major cause of bloat in cattle and should never be fed in large amounts to tortoises.

Spinach, beets, and Swiss chard have a high content of oxalate, which may bind calcium in the gastrointestinal tract, but they are nutritious as part of a balanced diet. All types of lettuces have a low mineral content; red leaf and romaine are the best of the lettuces but should still be fed less than other dark leafy greens. Frye[16] has seen goiters in Galapagos tortoises fed cabbage exclusively without sufficient dietary iodine. Again, if fed in moderation as part of a balanced diet, these vegetables are nutritious and will not cause problems.

<5% Fruits—Fruits tend to be mineral and protein poor but are a good source of carbohydrates and fiber. Tortoises readily consume fruits over other foods, so they need to be limited. Red- and yellow-foot tortoises are more frugivorous than other tortoises and should be offered more fruit, up to 20% of the entire ration. Tortoises eat grapes, apples, oranges, pears, prickly pear fruit, peaches, plums, nectarines, dates, all types of melons, strawberries, raspberries, bananas, mangos, and tomatoes.

High Protein Content Foods—"High-protein foods" is a descriptive term that should not be taken literally. Many fruits and vegetables also have a substantial protein content. Generally these foods are limited to once every 2 weeks in small amounts. Tortoises eat dry, maintenance low-fat dog food, pelleted parrot chows, tofu, various cereals (crisped rice, corn flakes, grape nuts, bran flakes, etc.), whole mice, baby mice, large-carnivore diets, and scrambled or hard boiled eggs (with shells). Dry chows should be soaked in lukewarm water for 15 to 30 minutes until softened. Some genera (*Kinixys*, *Chersina*, and *Manouria*) are more omnivorous and may benefit from small amounts of high-protein foods. It is widely assumed that high-protein foods promote rapid growth in young tortoises, which may result in pyramidal shell growth. These assumptions are controversial and remain unproven. The high protein, fat, and multivitamin content of these foods can be dangerous in excess and may promote hepatic lipidosis. But in moderation, as a very small portion of the diet, they are not likely to be harmful. Others feel tortoises should not have any of these foods and recommend an entirely vegetarian diet.

To make salad, rinse, chop, and mix two or three types of dark leafy greens, some thawed frozen mixed vegetables, sprouts, and whatever other vegetables are available. This mixture can be fed directly or stored in a large sealable container and refrigerated for up to 6 days. Before feeding, add freshly chopped fruits and occasionally (not more than twice a month) some high-protein foods. Put the salad on a flat board, piece of newspaper, or paper plate, or use plastic or metal plates or trays. Disposable feeding trays cut down on cleaning. Salad mixture that has been refrigerated should be allowed to come to room temperature for 30 to 60 minutes before feeding. **Feed as much variety as possible**!

Adults should be fed a minimum of three times per week and hatchlings daily. Every feeding, lightly dust food with calcium lactate, carbonate, citrate, or gluconate. Every 1 to 2 weeks lightly dust food with multivitamins (if vitamin-fortified foods are not present). If the tortoises are exposed to unfiltered sunlight, vitamin D supplements are not needed or desired.

Reproduction

Female tortoises must be in prime condition prior to egg production. This includes a well-balanced diet with adequate calcium. Small tortoises can be palpated in the inguinal fossa for eggs, but this is much more difficult in larger tortoises. A large female tortoise can cause excruciating pain to the forefinger foolhardy enough to be caught between her shell and rear leg. Eggs show up well on radiographs.

Gravid females feel heavier than normal and tend to be more active, often pacing in the cage. For nesting, areas are often selected that get the most sun or late afternoon sun. If the keeper is not present during egg laying, the nest can be easily missed. A definite sign that a female has been digging is dirt packed on her hindfeet and rear margins of shell. Some females may excavate several nests before actually laying eggs. Indoors one must provide a nesting substrate at least as deep as the female's carapace length. Oxytocin, at 2 to 10 IU/kg subcutaneously (SC) or intramuscularly (IM), in the rear legs, is effective in inducing oviposition within several hours in females reluctant to lay. The nest should be carefully excavated and eggs removed for incubation (see incubation section in chapter 1).

Neonatal care

Once the neonate has pipped the eggshell with its caruncle, or eggtooth, it will emerge from the shell within 1 to 4 days. During this time, the neonate's shell begins to unfold, facilitating yolk absorption. As the neonate's shell straightens and the tortoise begins to move, the eggshell breaks further.

Once out of the egg, the neonate may still have considerable yolk sac. The hatchling should be transferred to a container, such as a plastic shoe or sweater box, with clean moist paper towels. The yolk sac will be slowly absorbed over the next few days.

Once the yolk sac is fully absorbed and the umbilicus sealed, the hatchling can be transferred to a cage with previously mentioned substrates. Hatchlings usually begin feeding within 1 to 14 days of leaving the egg. Hatchlings are prone to dehydration; therefore shallow water bowls should constantly be available. Make sure the water bowl is shallow or the hatchling may overturn and drown. Plastic plant saucers work admirably for water bowls. An alternative is to soak neonates in shallow water three times a week. This option is less desirable in that invariably one occasionally forgets to soak tortoises.

Ultraviolet lights should be provided for 12 hours per day. A thermal gradient should be provided. Ambient temperature should not get colder than 24°C (75°F) at night and gradually warm to 30°C (85°F) during the day. Temperatures cooler than this are devastating to hatchling tortoises and can quickly lead to respiratory problems, anorexia, and death. Temperate young tortoises should be given a carefully controlled, shorter hibernation period or not hibernated at all for the first several years (see hibernation section in this chapter).

Hatchlings can be fed the previously described ration daily, finely chopped in a food processor. Hatchlings should develop a firm shell well within the first year. It is common for a clutch of siblings to have different growth rates. Smaller timid individuals may eventually need to be separated to ensure adequate nutrition.

Aquatic Turtle Care

Introduction

Aquatic turtles are popular pets, but this does not mean they are easy to care for. In fact, they can be among the most labor intensive of all reptiles to maintain. Inadequate care often results in problems for turtles. To treat these problems effectively, the veterinarian must be able to evaluate and correct captive care. Keep in mind that there are exceptions to most rules and there is no substitute for good information on the natural history of any aquatic turtle.

Taxonomy

The most common genera seen in the pet trade in the United States include *Trachemys* (sliders), *Chrysemys* (painted turtles), *Kinosternon* and *Sternotherus* (mud and musk turtles), *Graptemys* (map turtles), *Clemmys* (wood and pond turtles), *Apalone* (formerly *Trionyx*, soft shell turtles), *Pseudemys* (river cooters), *Chelydra* (common snapping turtles), *Malaclemys* (diamondback terrapins), *Macroclemys* (alligator snapping turtles), *Chelus* (matamatas), *Cuora* (Asiatic box turtles), *Chinemys* (Reeve's turtle), *Geoemyda* (leaf turtles), and *Platysternon* (big-headed turtles).

Housing

Housing requirements vary according to the size of the turtle and the number being kept. A variety of enclosures can be utilized, from glass aquariums, plastic cement mixing containers, stock watering tanks, and pond liners to elaborate outdoor ponds. Outdoor enclosures should have some shade available. Never place a plastic or glass aquarium in full sun, as it can easily overheat. A rule of thumb for minimum cage size is that the combined carapace size of all residents should not exceed 25% of the cage's floor surface area.[77] Floor surface area does not include any inaccessible areas that the turtle cannot rest on.

Water quality

Water laden with bacteria and nitrogenous wastes smells and can quickly infect turtle shells or kill turtles. Aquatic turtles should have little odor unless associated with feeding or musk glands. Turtle odor suggests a major water quality problem. Clean water is crucial to good health, and there are several means to ensure this.

Frequent full water changes are one method of keeping water clean. One can keep the water cleaner by feeding in a separate container, as most foods foul the water quickly. If the turtles are fed in their regular enclosure, the water should be changed within 12 hours of feeding messy foods. Initially some turtles may be reluctant to feed in the separate container, but they can be acclimated to this over time. Using the same water from the home container helps.

The frequency of water changes depends on the stocking density. For instance, for three or fewer 4-inch turtles, a 10-gallon aquarium should be changed two to three times per week and a 50-gallon aquarium once a week. It is easier when doing full water changes if no substrates are in the cage. Sand or gravel makes cleaning much more difficult. For smaller setups (10-gallon aquariums or less), one can carry the whole setup to a sink or bathtub for rinsing. Keep in mind that cleaning areas are a potential source of infectious bacteria, such as *Salmonella* (see *Salmonella* section in chapter 1). The 10-gallon storage container from Rubbermaid is easier to clean and more durable than a 10-gallon aquarium and is excellent for hatchlings.

For larger setups, one must drain the water. Portable electric submersible pumps can drain large volumes of water very quickly and make cleaning much less labor intensive. These pumps are designed to drain swimming pools or flooded basements and may be found in hardware stores or pool supply stores. The Little Giant Pump Company (Oklahoma City, OK) makes a very good one, called the "Water Wizard," model 5-MSP, for about $65.00. Alternatively, one can use a siphon to drain the water, but this requires much more time. If one has the luxury of floor drains, one can install drains in the bottom of the cage, attach a hose, and drain the cage by gravity. Refill larger setups through a hose (with a nozzle) attached to a faucet. Separate drainage and refill hoses make cleaning much more convenient. When using a hose to drain or refill a cage, be sure to secure the end of the hose carefully or inadvertent flooding will occur.

It is important to scrub and rinse the cage well periodically to remove residual bacterial growth on all sides. Abrupt changes in water temperature can kill turtles, so make sure the water temperature after cleaning is similar to what it was prior to cleaning. Thermometers facilitate this; with experience one can gauge this with one's hand. Dechlorination of the water is generally not necessary; chlorinated water may help keep bacterial levels down. Obviously, with biologic filtration systems, water must be dechlorinated. Young turtles and those not accustomed to chlorinated water initially squint their eyes and have difficulty eating but quickly acclimate.

A partial alternative to the laborious task of full water changes is biological or chemical filtration. Filtration can decrease the time interval required for partial to full water changes but should not completely eliminate them. The author's early impression of fish filtration systems, used with turtles, was that filtration simply did not work. However, our knowledge and the design of filtration systems for aquatic turtles have improved dramatically in the past few years (see Highfield[73] for a good review). Filtration is now desirable whenever feasible, especially for larger setups. Keep in mind that turtles produce considerably more solid fecal and urinary waste than fish. Most retail aquarium supply stores sell filters designed for biological breakdown of fish waste, not turtle waste. Even if the water looks clean, it can still have a great deal of nitrogenous waste in it. In general, select filters for turtles that are designed for large fish or high stocking densities. As with all filtration systems, good aeration of water (through airstones or water agitated by falling into the surface, such as with a waterfall) is important to support aerobic bacterial growth in biological filters. For small setups, internal submersible filters are gaining in popularity. The best filters for turtles are large biological or chemical filters, such as those designed for koi fish, rapid sand filters, and external canister filters. If the water level can be maintained within 8 inches of the top of the tank, power lifting hanging filters are less expensive and simpler to maintain than canister filters, but they are also much less effective because of lower flow rates and filtration surface area. Under-gravel filters need a deep gravel bed (7.5 cm or more), or the turtle may dig and expose the filter plate.[73] Once it is exposed, water will bypass most of the gravel as it follows the path of least resistance, and the benefits of biological filtration will be decreased. Foam rubber filters are essentially worthless. Disasters, such as die-offs, can result from poor water quality, particularly with low levels of oxygen saturation.

Water should be at least as deep as the width of the widest turtle's shell so that, if overturned, the turtle will be able to right itself and avoid drowning. Diamondback terrapins live in brackish water and require addition of two tablespoons of aquarium salt and mineral mix per gallon of water.

Temperature

Water, and air, must be warm; 24 to 28°C (75 to 82°F) is recommended for most species. An incandescent 50- to 150-watt light bulb, with reflector, directed toward the basking area will create a hot spot for basking. Alternatively, one can keep the room temperature within this range. Submersible aquarium heaters are ideal for warming water. Some species such as mud and musk turtles, common snapping turtles (not alligator snapping turtles), and Chinese big-headed turtles prefer it a little cooler.

Haul-out area

A dry "haul-out" area should be present so that turtles can crawl out of the water, dry off, and bask. Basking is a means of behavioral thermoregulation whereby turtles can achieve their preferred optimum body temperature. Basking areas can be as simple as a flat rock resting on submerged bricks or a cinder block. More elaborate platforms can be built into the cage above water level with access via a plastic ramp or piece of wood. One also can use floating pieces of cork, hardwood driftwood, or plastic floating platforms. Snapping turtles and Matamatas do not need basking areas.

Nesting areas

Nesting areas should be provided for adult females, even if adult males are not present. If a sufficient nest area is provided, dystocia may be avoided and oviposition stimulated. The Columbus Zoo has a prodigious aquatic turtle breeding program and believes that temporarily rigging a nesting area, or shifting a gravid female to a cage with a nesting area, is far less successful than keeping a nesting area present year-round.

The nesting area should be approximately four to five times larger than the carapace of the female. Nest medium should be slightly moist sand or potting soil and two times deeper than the length of the carapace. Nest area containers can be made from a large plastic trash can cut in half or a variety of smaller plastic containers. The nesting area can double as a basking area.

Feeding

Feed adults one to three times per week, hatchlings daily. **Feed as much variety as possible.** The majority of the diet should consist of whole animals such as mice, earthworms, slugs, snails, shrimp (with shells) and thawed frozen goldfish, guppies, trout, bait fish, and some smelt. Whole fish are better than gutted fish and can be fed chopped or whole. Most suppliers of feeder fish minimize their feeding to ensure good water quality in overcrowded setups. Ideally, fish should be well fed before being fed to turtles. Freezing for more than 3 days may eliminate transfer of some, but not all, parasites.[78] Goldfish can be frozen in ice cube trays to reduce freezer burn. Wild-caught sticklebacks and mosquito fish should not be fed because they are natural vectors for several serious parasites. Avoid large quantities of oil-laden species such as mackerel and to a lesser extent smelt and goldfish, which are known to induce steatitis. Smelt can have high levels of thiaminase (especially after freezing), which can induce thiamine or vitamin B_1 deficiency if fed exclusively. If fed in moderation, as part of a balanced diet, frozen fish should not cause any problems (see the chapter on caimans for more information).

Most aquatic turtles readily consume mice, from pinkies to chopped skinned adults. Older mice have more mineralized bone and are an outstanding source of calcium and phosphorus for shell growth. Mouse liver is also a good source of vitamin A. A variety of insects (crickets, waxworms, mealworms, flies, moths, and grasshoppers) in moderation are also good. Be aware that insects are calcium deficient (see the section on feeding insectivorous reptiles and amphibians in chapter 4). Earthworms are widely available and nutritious; small turtles often need them chopped. Snails and slugs can also be fed.

Commercial diets can provide a smaller portion of the diet and should be soaked until soft before offering them to the turtle. A variety have been used including Trout, Catfish or Shrimp Chow (Ralston Purina), Hikari Chichlid Gold pelleted fish food (Kyorin Co.), Reptomin Floating Food Sticks (Tetra), Tender Vittles or Happy Cat semimoist cat foods (Ralston Purina), Gaines Burger semimoist dog food (Gaines), and various commercial turtle diets. Patience and persistence are required with commercial diets because acceptance can take several weeks. Check the ingredients; desiccated insects are nutritionally inadequate and should not be fed.

Small amounts of lean raw beef, liver, gizzards, or chicken can occasionally be fed but are severely calcium deficient unless bone is present. Hamburger is not recommended because it is calcium deficient and the high fat content leaves a greasy film on the surface of the water.

Many sliders and pond turtles become more herbivorous as they reach mature size and grow less rapidly. One can gradually increase dark leafy greens (kale, romaine lettuce, cabbage, watercress, endive, bok choy, escarole, spinach), duckweed, algae, and fruits (apples, oranges, carrot, grapes, melons, bananas) for these species.

Neonatal care

Hatchling aquatic turtles can be a challenge to raise. Avoid crowding neonate turtles. A 10-gallon plastic storage container works well for young turtles because it is easily cleaned and the nontransparent sides may offer additional security. Hatchlings may be shy and scramble for cover at your approach and can be reluctant to feed. Provide hatchlings with cover to retreat under, such as floating pieces of cork, clay flower-pot pieces, plastic leaves (large enough that they cannot be ingested), or a small board or flat rock over bricks. Be certain that cage props are stable so that they do not shift, trap young turtles underwater, and drown them.

To coerce young turtles to feed, try small live insects such as 2-week-old crickets, mealworms, waxworms, chopped pink mice, or small chopped earthworms. As the hatchlings begin to feed with more vigor, try a wider variety of foods. As soon as possible, try to get them eating finely chopped adult mice, guppies, or small goldfish, all good sources of bone. Hikari Chichlid Gold pelleted fish food and trout chow are good because the pellets come in a wide variety of sizes that can be increased as the turtle grows. UV lights, proper temperature, and a wide variety of foods are important to prevent metabolic bone disease and ensure proper growth.

As much variety as possible is recommended to ensure a healthy diet for aquatic turtles. If a balanced diet with whole mice is provided, multivitamin and mineral supplementation is not required and could be detrimental in the long run. Encourage owners to experiment with their turtles. Reassure them that dietary changes are important, but acceptance on the part of the turtle can take time (weeks to months). The owner should not be discouraged if novel items are tasted and spit out initially; it can take weeks for turtles to accept new foods.

Species interactions

Some turtle species, such as snapping turtles, large soft shell turtles, mud and musk turtles, and big-headed turtles, are aggressive toward other turtles. These species can cause severe lacerations or kill other species and should be kept only with others of the same species and size. Cannibalism is known to occur in the Chelydridae, Emydidae, Kinosternidae, and Trionychidae. In addition, many aquatic turtles can be asymptomatic carriers of *Entamoeba invadens,* which can cause serious gastrointestinal disease in other reptiles.

Basic Medical Techniques for Turtles, Tortoises, and Terrapins

Handling

Handle chelonians by their shells, not their appendages. Certain species (soft-shell, snapping, big-headed, mud and musk turtles) are notorious biters. Large turtles should never be handled by the tail; instead, grab the rear or side portions of the carapace. Do not rotate large tortoises for fear of intestinal torsion. The main dangers in handling chelonians are from bites, scratches, urination, musk glands, and, in large chelonians, crushing a finger or hand against the inner shell.

Physical examination

When performing the physical exam, start at the head. Extend the head by getting both front legs out and then applying slow, steady traction to the head. Great strength is not required. Once the head is out far enough, grasp it from above just caudal to the skull. This prevents the turtle from retracting its head back into the shell. For most chelonians weighing more than 1 kg (unless very tame) chemical restraint is needed, such as 50 mg/kg ketamine IM or 10 mg/kg Telazol. Examine the oral cavity. Steady traction on the lower jaw will open it enough for a good look around or placement of a mouth speculum. Look for obvious lesions, pallor, ulcers, discharge from the glottis or internal nares, or flukes. Examine the external nares for abnormal discharge and eyes for blepharoedema. Ocular discharge is normal in some species, such as red- and yellow-footed tortoises, but abnormal in most. Nasal discharge is generally abnormal. Auscultate over the nares with the open bell of a good-quality cardiac or pediatric stethoscope and listen to a few breaths. Clicks, squeaks, rales, and so on are abnormal. Open-mouthed breathing is abnormal unless it is a threat display. Temporal muscle atrophy is common with extreme cachexia. Before releasing the head palpate the middle ear cavities; they should be slightly concave with nothing palpable. Check the eustachian tubes for any discharge from the middle ears. Release the head and examine all legs and fossae for swellings or myiasis. Eggs, cystic calculi, or abdominal masses are palpable anterior or medial to the inguinal fossae with slow lateral rocking. Weigh small turtles with a gram scale, turtles over 2.5 kg are best weighed on a conventional small-animal scale. Measure straight carapace length with calipers and a ruler for determination of the weight-to-length value (see the next section on weight evaluation). Aquatic turtles should be evaluated in water deep enough for them to float. They should float levelly from side to side but not front to back. Determine the sex to complete the medical history and satisfy the owner's curiosity. In many male turtles the cloaca is beyond the rear carapacial shell margins (figure 7). Mature males tend to have longer tails (figure 7) and sometimes a concave plastron. Head, eye, or body coloration is usually more pronounced in males (figures 8 and 9) and claws are occasionally dimorphic. For example, slider males have longer front nails and female leopard tortoises have longer rear nails.

Weight evaluation

With experience, most veterinarians become good judges of whether a turtle is over- or underweight. An underweight turtle feels light for its shell size. However, as turtles become larger it becomes increasingly difficult to evaluate body weight objectively because the shell is often quite heavy itself. The late Oliphant F. Jackson plotted body weight versus length for captive Mediterranean tortoises, *Testudo graeca* and *T. hermanni*.[79] Dr. Jackson found that for a given carapace length there was a normal or healthy body weight and sick tortoises were often well below this weight (or well above if obese). This relationship (called Jackson's ratio) has been clinically useful for European veterinarians working with these species. Jackson's ratio has also been listed for desert tortoises.[80] Unfortunately, growth curves are fairly species specific. Jackson and Lawrence[81] reported that weight-to-length relationships were not useful for terrapins (aquatic turtles), and Jacobson et al.[82] cautioned against using Jackson's ratio as a sole criterion for evaluating the health of desert tortoises. Donoghue[83] analyzed weight-to-length data for 76 tortoises representing 11 species and derived the equation: body weight = 0.191(SCL^3), where SCL^3 is straight carapace length, in centimeters, cubed. This equation allows one to calculate whether a given tortoise is above or below its estimated weight, but keep in mind that a sick animal may still be within normal weight.

Venipuncture

Chelonians are bled from several different sites, depending on personal preference and the size of the patient. For turtles weighing 50 g or less, cardiocentesis is most practical. Localization of the heart with a Doppler detector or ultrasonography is useful, but keep in mind that the heart moves slightly forward with the head extended. In general, the heart is dorsal or just anterior to the intersection of humeral and abdominal scutes but it can vary between individuals and species. After sterile preparation of the shell, a 25-gauge needle is used to pierce the shell with the patient in dorsal recumbency so that the needle does not prematurely puncture the heart. The patient is then reoriented, with the plastron ventrally, and a smaller gauge needle is used for cardiac puncture, up from below the heart, through the guide hole. This position stabilizes the heart in better contact with the plastron and increases the probability of piercing such a small organ. Afterward, a drop of tissue adhesive, sterile bone wax, or epoxy closes the hole.

In larger turtles a variety of other sites, such as the dorsal coccygeal vein, radiohumeral or femoral venous plexus, jugular vein, or clipping a nail bed, are accessible and less invasive. One study found no differences in red blood cell counts, packed cell volumes, or hemoglobin concentrations between the dorsal coccygeal vein and clipped nail beds in Mediterranean tortoises.[84] However, if the foot is squeezed to milk blood out, there may be a drop in the red blood cell count, packed cell volume, and hemoglobin concentration. In contrast, blood samples collected from the postoccipital venous plexus (POVP) had significantly lower hematological and plasma biochemistry values than those obtained from the jugular vein in desert tortoises.[85] Lymph dilution at the POVP was believed to be responsible. The same was not found to be true for blood versus lymph dilute plasma biochemical values in red-eared sliders except for total protein and potassium.[86] Whenever possible, blood should be obtained from the jugular vein or underlying carotid artery. In giant tortoises nail bed hemostasis can be extremely difficult and is best avoided. Light chemical restraint greatly assists venipuncture of timid chelonians.

The dorsal coccygeal vein runs on the *dorsal* midline above the coccygeal vertebrae. This site is often useful in turtles too small to bleed through the jugular vein. The coccygeal vertebrae lack dorsal spinous processes. A small gauge needle is inserted perpendicular to the tail surface in the anterior third of the tail; the vein tends to be very superficial.

Another site, developed in sea turtles[87] but also useful in small turtles, is the dorsal cervical sinuses on either side of midline along the neck. Turtles should be restrained with the head held down and fully extended (to fill the sinuses). A needle is inserted, perpendicular to the dorsal neck, 0.5 to 1 cm lateral from the dorsal cervical midline, to a depth of 0.5 to 3 cm depending on the turtles' size. An angled table with a slot in front for withdrawing the turtle's head facilitates unassisted sampling.

A large venous plexus caudal to the radiohumeral joint is useful in turtles over 1 kg and for repeated blood collections. To approach this sinus, extend the front leg and palpate the prominent tendon on the back side of the leg. Insert the needle just dorsal or ventral to the tendon, perpendicular to the skin and angling toward the caudomedial radiohumeral joint with slight plunger pressure (figure 10). The plexus lies just posterior to the joint up to half the distance from the posterior skin surface. A similar plexus exists near the distal caudal femur and is useful in smaller turtles.

The preferred site in larger chelonians is the jugular vein (figure 11). To approach this vein, have someone restrain the turtle in lateral recumbency, with slight pressure across the base of the neck and the ipsilateral front leg extended. The phlebotomist extends and lowers the head with one hand and draws with the other. Slightly bending the needle assists venipuncture. A 23- to 25-gauge butterfly catheter, with the cap removed, permits easier blood flow and allows one to maintain patency for collection of larger volumes of blood.[88] The jugular vein is usually visible laterally along a line caudal or just dorsal to a line from the angle of mandible in desert tortoises and box turtles. Some of the neck muscles may be mistaken for the vein and it may take a bit of positioning and palpating to be sure of the jugular veins position. Apply light pressure to the jugular vein (or carotid artery) for 3 to 5 minutes after venipuncture to avoid hematoma formation.[88] In *Testudo* and many cryptodiran aquatic turtles the jugular generally cannot be visualized.

Fluid administration

There are numerous routes of fluid administration for chelonians; often a combination of routes is efficacious.

Soaking—Dehydrated chelonians take up water well through the cloaca and by drinking if allowed to soak in shallow lukewarm water for 8 to 12 hours. Water should be no more than chin deep. If the chelonian is not seriously dehydrated, this is generally the author's initial approach.

Enteral—Stomach tubing is feasible in weak chelonians but is a chore in stronger patients. See the sections on stomach tubing and esophagostomy tube placement later in this chapter.

Subcutaneous—Small volumes can be given under the finely scaled skin on the limbs. Avoid thickly scaled areas, which are difficult to pass a needle through. Avoid the coelomic cavity as well (see following).

Epicoelomic—In a chelonian that is completely retracted into its shell and difficult to coerce out, epicoelomic fluids are easier to administer than subcutaneous or intracoelomic fluids. The epicoelomic space is the potential space above the plastron and below the pectoral muscles and coelom. A 1- to 1.5-inch needle is inserted ventral to the scapulohumeral joint, parallel and just dorsal to the plastron, and directed caudally toward the opposite hind leg. There should be little resistance to fluid administration if epicoelomic and not intramuscular. Another advantage of this site is that no vital organs can be compromised under the pectoral muscles.

Intracoelomic—This author avoids intracoelomic fluids because they may compromise the lung space within the rigid shell, and lungs are easily perforated (especially if the needle is directed anteriomedially in the dorsal half of the inguinal fossa), or a distended urinary bladder may be punctured. Many practitioners do use intracoelomic fluids safely, the key is to inject fluids caudally in the ventral inguinal fossa.

Rates—Maintenance fluid volumes have empirically been dosed at 15 (large reptiles) to 25 (small reptiles) ml/kg/day divided q 12–24 hr. For severe dehydration 40 ml/kg/day divided q 12 hr has been used in tortoises.[89]

Types—Equal parts of 5% dextrose or 0.45% NaCl (if the patient is hyperglycemic), mixed with nonlactated crystalloid solutions (such as Normo-Sol-R, Ceva Labe, Overland Park, KS, or Plasma-Lyte, Baxter Health Care, Deerfield, IL), are recommended for rehydrating reptiles.[90] Fluids should be warmed to the preferred body temperature for the given species or 80°F. Other crystalloid fluids (0.9% NaCl or lactated Ringer's solution) have been used successfully.

Stomach tubing

Tube feeding chelonians is generally a two-person procedure. It is easier to pass a tube down the esophagus with the neck extended. With the head and neck extended and the turtle held vertically, the maxilla is opened and a speculum inserted. Lubricate the tip of the feeding tube and pass it down the esophagus (avoid the glottis at the base of the tongue) to the left center of the plastron where the stomach lies. Slight resistance is usually felt as the tube passes through the gastroesophageal sphincter. Tube feed 15 to 25 ml/kg of the tube feeding formula slowly over a minute or so. Stop and remove the tube if the formula refluxes up the esophagus. Keep the neck extended and the turtle vertical for a minute after tube feeding. If the tube was not passed deep enough into the stomach, the tube feeding formula will reflux up the esophagus. Typically tube feeding is every other day to every third or fourth day (the longer interval with longer therapy). On alternate days, tube-feed water or balanced electrolytes. Monitor fecal output as one measure of how often to tube feed.

A variety of formulas have been used for tube feeding in the past. For several years the author had good success in box turtles with Emeraid II (LaFaber Co., Odell, IL) and in aquatic turtles with A/D (Science Diet, Topeka, KS). The reader is referred to a review of reptile nutrition suggesting several more suitable liquid enterals for use with different reptiles and disease conditions.[80] Science Diet A/D is purine rich and is probably not good for dehydrated reptiles.[80]

Esophagostomy tube placement

Long-term enteral support in chelonians is simplified by placing a red rubber catheter through the skin, at the base of the neck, into the esophagus and then into the stomach. The tube should be placed through the turtle's right neck, to minimize tube bending as the esophagus courses to the turtle's left to meet the stomach. Direct hemostats through the mouth as far caudally as feasible and then incise over the hemostat tips ventrolaterally near the base of the neck. The tube is placed caudally to minimize tube movement with neck movement and prevent the leg from pawing at it. Take care to avoid large vessels in the neck. Grab the tube tip with the hemostats, retract it into the esophagus, and then redirect the tube posteriorly into the stomach (midplastron level). The tube may be secured with an interlocking Chinese fingertrap pattern or taped and sutured to the skin. Cap and flush the tube with water after each use; excess tube can be taped to the carapace.

Tracheal wash

Radiographic evaluation of lung fields is useful for localizing sites of respiratory problems. There are several approaches to a lung wash. Trephination of the lungs is one invasive technique. As an alternative, sterile orthopedic wire can be used to curve an appropriately sized red rubber catheter to cannulate the desired mainstem bronchi. Infuse 1 to 5 ml/kg sterile saline and then carefully rock the patient before withdrawing saline. A percutaneous lung wash is also practical through the inguinal fossa.[91] An appropriate-sized needle can be directed toward the lesion, which is flushed with a similar volume of sterile saline.

Gastric and cloacal wash

Washes are a good means of detecting protozoal problems. Ball tip stainless steel gavage tubes can be used to collect small volumes of infused 0.9% NaCl. Immediately examine floating particulate matter for protozoans. A colonic surface biopsy can be obtained via "cloacal wash."

Diseases of Turtles, Tortoises, and Terrapins

Hypovitaminosis A

Chelonians are prone to dietary deficiencies of vitamin A. It is the most common problem of box turtles seen in private veterinary practice.[92] Clinical signs include blepharoedema, usually with (in chronic cases) or without (in early cases) solid whitish-yellow cellular debris underneath the eyelids, lethargy, anorexia, weight loss, and nasal or ocular discharge (figure 12). Anorexia is thought to result from visual impairment.

Treatment of hypovitaminosis A varies. The author prefers 2000 IU/kg body weight Aquasol A parenteral SC in the front leg once every 7 to 14 days for two to four treatments. Typical dosages are 0.01 to 0.02 ml per week. Ocular improvement takes 2 to 6 weeks, depending on the severity of presenting signs; be sure to mention this to owners.

Cellular debris under the eyelids can be removed carefully with a smooth-edged blunt probe and digital pressure. Ophthalmic antibiotic ointments or solutions are warranted if secondary infection is present, but many infections resolve spontaneously once hypovitaminosis is corrected. If both globes are eviscerated, the turtle has a poor prognosis for long-term survival.

Warm shallow water soaks daily for several hours are beneficial. Once the turtle's eyelids open, encourage it to eat vitamin A–rich foods. If the turtle is severely underweight, it can be tube fed with avian hand-feeding formulas after dehydration has been corrected. Obviously, long-term treatment requires improved nutrition. See Elkan and Zwart[93] for detailed pathogenesis and Boyer[94] for more information.

Hypervitaminosis A is also possible given the concentrated forms of vitamin A available, small size of many patients, and wide dosage ranges in the literature.[95] Frye[12] described iatrogenic hypervitaminosis as initially causing dry, flaky skin (xeroderma). Within a few days, erythematous areas spread all over the skin. In these areas, the epidermis detaches from the underlying dermis, forming moist blisters, within 2 to 3 weeks of overdosage. The epidermal blisters then slough by 3 to 4 weeks, exposing a moist, reddened, underlying dermis (figure 13) and, in some areas, underlying muscle.[12,95] Supportive care consists of topical antibiotics on exposed dermis, parenteral fluids, and shallow warm water (24 to 27°C [75 to 80°F]) soaks for several hours daily.

Vitamin A should not be used indiscriminately in chelonians.[12] If dietary history and clinical signs suggest a deficiency, vitamin A should be dosed carefully and given for no more than four treatments (see hypovitaminosis A). Oral supplementation has a much greater margin of safety than injection.[12]

Upper respiratory tract infections

Upper respiratory tract infections are common in captive tortoises and turtles and have devastated native populations of desert tortoises, *Gopherus agassizii*. Left untreated, upper respiratory tract infections slowly debilitate chelonians. In wild chelonians death may take a year, but in captivity tortoises may survive for years.[96] Owners often need to be convinced of the severity of this disease as their chelonian may have had symptoms for years. Clinical signs of upper respiratory tract disease (URTD) include clear to colored discharge or bubbling from the nares (figure14), decreased to no appetite, and lethargy. Other more subtle signs may be ocular discharge, conjunctivitis, palpebral edema, sunken eyes (if dehydrated), dull coloration, and weight loss. Nasal discharge is best detected after pushing the tortoise's head straight back into its shell. Any nasal discharge is abnormal, except if the turtle or tortoise has just been drinking. If the nares are occluded, discharge from the nares may not be detectable. Prolonged nasal discharge results in erosion of the nares and formation of ventral grooves. Jacobson et al.[96] reported URTD in a wide variety of *Gopherus* and *Geochelone* and one wonders if this is not the same disease as runny nose syndrome in *Testudo*.[96,97]

Many other diseases can cause similar symptoms. Vitamin A deficiency can disrupt the epithelial lining of the nasal passages and predispose the turtle to secondary bacterial infections that result in nasal discharge. However, vitamin A deficiency typically causes palpebral swelling as well. An inhaled foreign body, such as a foxtail or grass awn lodged in the nasal cavity, would also produce nasal discharge. Excess salivation, heavy nematode loads, and inhaled irritants, such as pollen or dust, can also produce nasal discharge.

Mycoplasma agassizii is believed to be the primary causative agent.[96,98] A variety of other bacteria, particularly aerobic gram negatives, may also be present and may secondarily contribute to URTD. Pathogenesis is not well understood but may involve malnutrition, immunosuppression, and bacterial colonization.[96] An enzyme-linked immunosorbent assay (ELISA) is available through the University of Florida to determine whether tortoises have antibody to *Mycoplasma*. Bacterial culture for *Mycoplasma* is not recommended as a screening or diagnostic test because of low sensitivity and notorious difficulties in culturing *Mycoplasma*.

Mycoplasma is thought to spread from tortoise to tortoise through nasal exudates, directly or indirectly. Upper respiratory tract disease is extremely contagious among tortoises. Symptomatic chelonians should be immediately separated and asymptomatic chelonians in contact watched closely for nasal discharge. Healthy chelonians should not be in contact with affected animals even after recovery (unless they were previously housed together). Warn owners always to work with sick chelonians after healthy chelonians have been serviced, avoid sharing water bowls between cages or groups, and avoid mixing groups or species of chelonians indiscriminately. New turtles should be quarantined away from established stock for a minimum of 3 months. *Mycoplasma* is not vertically transmitted, which means that symptomatic or seropositive chelonians can produce healthy hatchlings if the hatchlings are reared separately.

Treatment consists of 3 to 6 weeks of enrofloxacin (Baytril, Haver Mobay) at 5 mg/kg q 24 hr in the soft skin of the front half of the chelonian. Nasal cavity flushes with antibiotics are very important to remove accumulated cellular debris and get antibiotics into the problem area (the nasal sinus). Jacobson[98] recommends flushing each nare with 0.5 ml of a 1:10 dilution of enrofloxacin and saline daily (for large groups go every third day) for one month. It is difficult to flush the nares when the turtle or tortoise has withdrawn its head into the shell. One trick for avoiding this is to place the larger end of an open-ended syringe case down to the nares before the turtle or tortoise withdraws its head. The syringe case can then be pushed in farther as the chelonian withdraws its head and legs. One then has access to the nares, through the syringe case, even with the head withdrawn.

If the turtle continues to eat or maintains good body weight, force feeding is not required. Progressive weight loss, sunken eyes, and weakness are indications for force feeding. In rare cases vitamin A injections may help, especially if dietary history and clinical signs (such as swollen eyelids) support a vitamin A deficiency. Vitamin A deficiency was implicated in the past, but current research does not appear to support this theory.[96]

Respiratory tract infections are a common sequel to chilling of chelonians. Another very important aspect of treatment is warming up the chelonian to its preferred optimum. Affected animals that recover seem to remain carriers and may have periodic relapses, especially with suboptimal environmental conditions, such as in winter. Relapses also respond well to treatment. Long-standing cases with severe nasal cavity damage may be less responsive to treatment. As URTD is so prevalent in captive chelonian collections, veterinarians should advise owners in no uncertain terms not to release captive tortoises, even if apparently healthy, into wild tortoise populations, even if the captives were once wild caught themselves.

Lower respiratory tract infections

The simple respiratory anatomy of chelonians makes them susceptible to lower respiratory tract infections. Squamous metaplasia from hypovitaminosis A may be an underlying predisposing factor. A wide variety of aerobic gram-negative and anaerobic bacteria can be recovered from respiratory tract infections. Viruses morphologically similar to herpes virus were associated with necrotizing glossitis and stomatitis and death in tortoises.[99–101] Fungal pneumonias have also been reported. *Mycoplasma* has not been documented as a lower respiratory pathogen in turtles, but given its pulmonary proclivity in other species one suspects it may be involved.

Early signs of lower respiratory tract infection can be easily overlooked. Often the chelonian is less active or stationary, eats less, and may have lost weight. As respiratory disease progresses, moist respiratory sounds, or gurgling, become evident. Nasal discharge is variable. Nasal discharge may be present if there is concurrent upper respiratory tract infection, but as the glottis is not contiguous with the internal nares, it is often absent. Severe cases have sunken eyes and are obviously dyspneic. They may breathe through their mouth if the nares are clogged, extend their neck to breathe, or pump their head and legs slowly while breathing. A click or squeak associated with respiration may be audible in aquatic turtles. Aquatic turtles also list laterally in water as the affected lung accumulates material and becomes less buoyant (figure 15).

Clinical signs are generally diagnostic. Radiographs, especially horizontal craniocaudal views, and lung washes for bacterial culture and sensitivity testing, as well as cytology, are important diagnostically (see the section on tracheal wash earlier in this chapter).

Abscesses

Shell abscesses and skin infections are prevalent among aquatic turtles in overcrowded or unsanitary conditions. Shell abscesses manifest as soft fluid-filled whitish or yellowish areas under the scutes with petechial to ecchymotic hemorrhages peripherally. A foul odor is often present, and owners are surprised to learn that captive aquatic turtles are typically odorless. The underlying bone is usually infected, and truly severe infections can penetrate the coelom. Bacteria are generally the culprits, although fungal infections are occasionally encountered. Most shell abscesses respond well to thorough debridement of infected scutes and bone under anesthesia and daily scrubbing with chlorhexidine scrub (Nolvasan wound cleanser, Fort Dodge). Water should be changed daily during treatment and water quality improved for long-term prevention. The debrided shell is left to granulate in, permanent scarring of the shell results. Systemic antibiotics are generally not needed unless bone is heavily involved. Shell abscesses are less common among terrestrial chelonians.

Middle ear infections

Box turtles and occasionally aquatic turtles are prone to infections of the middle ear cavity. Advanced cases are presented with unilateral or bilateral bulging of the tympanic membrane (figure 16). Solid cellular debris extends caudal to the tympanic membrane within the middle ear cavity. Ascending infections through the eustachian tubes may be the source of infection.[81,102] Once the turtle is anesthetized, treatment consists of incising along the ventral tympanic membrane rim from three to nine o'clock to allow good access to the middle ear cavity. Cellular debris is then curetted and the middle ear cavity is thoroughly flushed for several days postoperatively. Flushing is particularly important to remove all solid cellular debris. Hemorrhage is generally not a problem but can be controlled with light pressure or chemical cautery. Antibiotic ointments are recommended, as well as systemic antibiotics. Anorexia is prevalent with advanced cases. Even severe cases respond well to treatment; recurrence is not uncommon.

Winter anorexia

Almost all box turtles in the pet trade are wild-caught adults accustomed to hibernating. A typical scenario is the turtle whose appetite slowly declines in September and ceases in October and who presents in early winter for anorexia and signs of hypovitaminosis A. Winter is a particularly inappropriate time to purchase box turtles.

Treatment for winter anorexia primarily involves improved husbandry. The turtles should be exposed to an ultraviolet light photoperiod of 12 hours light per day. Increase the photoperiod by ½ hour per week until 14 hours of light per day is achieved. Set the cage up in a closet or a room without windows so that the outdoor photoperiod does not interfere with the artificial photoperiod. The increasing day length often stimulates appetite within 2 to 6 weeks. Ambient temperature should be warm (24 to 29°C [75 to 85°F]) and hypovitaminosis A and respiratory tract infections treated if present. If the turtle appears healthy initially hibernation is the best option (see hibernation section in this chapter).

Shell trauma and repair

Shell fractures often arise after encounter with lawnmowers, automobiles, dogs (figure 6), other vertebrate predators, and large hoofed stock and after falls. Involved repair of the shell should not be attempted until the patient is stable and shell fractures are clean. If the coelom is exposed, adhesive bandages with plastic backing or Saran Wrap® can be taped in place for an airtight seal to prevent desiccation. Turtles do not have a diaphragm, and inspiration is not heavily dependent on negative pressure; therefore, open fractures that expose the lungs seldom impair respiration.[12,103] Scrub the wounds daily with chlorhexidine (Nolvasan wound cleanser, Fort Dodge) or dilute tamed iodine for about a week before applying a fiberglass epoxy patch.

Once the damaged shell is cleaned and infection eliminated, fiberglass patches interlaced with 5-minute epoxy provide a strong, durable, waterproof patch to allow the shell to heal.[12,104] Be sure to use clear 5-minute epoxy, not quick-set, 20-minute, or regular epoxy. Clear epoxy allows one to monitor the fracture site visually over time. Anesthesia is recommended to ease application and better set fractures. Ophthalmic ointment is important to prevent corneal damage by the epoxy fumes. One final cleaning of the entire shell and fracture site with chlorhexidine scrub followed by flushing with sterile saline is recommended. Fracture edges should be reduced as much as possible; orthopedic wire can close large gaps, and collapsed shell portions should be elevated if possible. Clean the shell edges outside the fracture site with acetone to improve epoxy adhesion. Fiberglass patches (from boat or automobile repair kits available in most hardware stores) can be cut to the needed shape and autoclaved. Mix 5-minute epoxy, quickly apply it outside the wound edges, and apply the first fiberglass patch. Then lightly coat the patch with epoxy and repeat with one or two more layers. Be sure the epoxy does not seep into the fracture site as it will severely inhibit or prevent healing; antibiotic ointment in the fracture helps keep epoxy out. As the epoxy is worked into the fiberglass patch, the patch should become translucent (except perhaps directly over the fracture). It is essential that the patch be air- and watertight when finished to prevent opportunistic infections. Fracture sites difficult to patch, such as the skin and shell interface, can be sealed with clear silicon cement (the same type used for aquarium repair). Once finished, a light spraying of vegetable oil pan coating (such as PAM®) or a petroleum based ointment will eliminate the epoxy's tackiness immediately.[12] The patch should be left on until the shell heals, which can take 6 to 24 months.

Some veterinarians feel that shell fractures are better managed as open wounds, with cerclage wire and small epoxy patches for stabilization, and wet to dry bandages covering the majority of the wound.[105] A major disadvantage of this method is that bandages need to be changed for weeks to months before the shell seals with granulation tissue.

Ectoparasites

Ectoparasites most commonly include ticks in tortoises, leeches in aquatic turtles, and maggots in box turtles. Chelonians are rarely plagued by mites. Ticks are easily removed with hemostats, and salt works well to remove leeches. Cistudinomyia (formerly Sarcophaga) maggots are prevalent among box turtles, especially in the inguinal and axillary fossa, and have also been seen in tortoises and aquatic turtles. Flies deposit first-instar larvae on skin, which proceed to penetrate folds or wounds.[106] Larvae form subcutaneous cysts with an air hole on the surface of the turtle's skin lined with black material (figure 17). Usually there are several maggots per cyst and several cysts per turtle. Cysts rarely penetrate the coelom. Treatment consists of carefully removing maggots (under anesthesia), with hemostats, through the air hole (which may need to be slightly enlarged). Palpation is essential to be sure all maggots are removed; then flush the cysts well. After removing all maggots, the cysts should be flushed with a 1:30 dilution of chlorhexidine and saline. Box turtles generally recover well. Treatment should not be directed towards killing maggots and leaving them in situ.

Cystic calculi

Desert tortoises are prone to uric acid and ammonium acid urate cystic calculi. Tortoises may be asymptomatic or suffer from anorexia, lethargy, constipation, weakness of the rear legs, dystocia, or nasal discharge.[107] Diagnosis is possible with careful inguinal fossa palpation or radiographs (figure 18). The larger size of the right liver lobe than the left is thought to be the reason for the predominance of stones in the left lobe of the bladder.[108] Large tortoises can be difficult to palpate if timid. Treatment consists of celiotomy and cystotomy, antibiotics, and fluids. Anorexia for several weeks postoperatively is to be expected, and adequate hydration should be maintained. Consider nutritional support via stomach tubing or a esophagostomy tube if the turtle is underweight. Be sure the stone has not passed from the bladder to the cloaca, as cloacal stones are not accessible through a plastronal celiotomy. Cloacal stones appear within the pelvis on dorsoventral radiographs. Cloacal stones can be broken down and extracted percloacally.

Penile prolapse

Prolapse of the penis can occur secondary to metabolic bone disease (figure 19); constipation; impaction of the cloaca with urates; neurogenic defects in the penis retractor apparatus, cloacal vent, or anal sphincter muscles; bacterial, parasitic, or fungal infections of the superficial tissue; irritation and/or desiccation of the penis by substrates while attempting to breed; or trauma caused by breeding or cagemates.[12,102,109] Most owners are surprised to learn that such a large purplish or blackish mass protruding from the cloaca is the penis (turtles have a relatively large penis). If discovered early enough, the penis can be cleaned off, lubricated with an antibiotic ointment, and forced back into the cloaca. A pursestring suture around the cloaca is advisable for 2 to 3 weeks. If the penis is swollen after cleaning, soaking it in 50% dextrose may reduce edema enough that it may be replaced; if not, anesthetise the turtle and replace the penis or surgically enlarge the vent.[12] Many cases reprolapse. If the penis is necrotic or desiccated, amputation is necessary. Under anesthesia, double-ligate the base of the penis with two absorbable vertical mattress sutures and then amputate the distal penis.[12,109] This has no effect on the turtle's ability to urinate, as urinary products are deposited from the ureters directly into the urodeum and cloaca.[12] Be sure to distinguish a prolapsed penis from a prolapsed cloaca, intestine, or urinary bladder.[12]

Egg retention

Chelonians often fail to lay eggs if not provided with a suitable nesting substrate or soil to dig down into. Chelonians should ideally be able to excavate to a depth equal to the length of their carapace. A sure way to promote egg retention is to move an outdoor female indoors, especially if she had already laid several earlier clutches outdoors. Hypovitaminosis A, egg yolk celoemitis, cystic or cloacal calculi, malnutrition, dehydration, and metabolic bone disease are other common causes of egg retention. Clinical signs include anorexia, lethargy or increased pacing, excavating nests without depositing eggs (several false nests may be a normal part of egg laying), straining to pass eggs, or hemorrhagic discharge from the cloaca.[110] Palpation of the inguinal fossa can detect the presence but not the number of eggs. Radiographs determine how many eggs are present; rule out any physical causes of egg retention, such as overly large, anomalous, or fractured eggs, thickened or roughened eggshells, or masses impinging on the terminal oviducts or pelvic inlet[12]; and, most importantly, allow one to choose medical versus surgical management early on.[111] A chemistry panel may also yield insight into the female's condition. Evaluation of cloacal or perhaps transceloemic aspirates can be useful in detecting egg yolk celomitis, which has a poor prognosis. Laparoscopy, if available, is also extremely useful.

If radiographs appear normal, the female should be given 100 mg/kg 10% calcium gluconate intracoelomically, placed in shallow lukewarm water if dehydrated or a suitable nesting substrate, and kept at the preferred optimal temperature range with minimal disturbance. Once rehydrated (usually 12 to 24 hours later), consider 1 to 10 IU oxytocin/kg IM in the rear leg if the female has not produced eggs. Oxytocin generally results in oviposition within several hours. If there is no response after several injections, consider the female's overall condition in terms of the advisability of celiotomy versus giving the female more time. Healthy, alert females that are eating well often lay eggs if given sufficient time. In contrast one three-toed box turtle (*Terrapene carolina triunguis*) that did not respond to repeated oxytocin injections and loosened soil in an outdoor nesting pen was found to have a pyometra during celiotomy. After ovariosalpingotomy, she did well.[112]

If medical management fails or is not an option, consider plastral celiotomy or osteotomy. Sterile surgery should be observed; this often requires a little improvisation. High-speed dental, orthopedic, and dremel tools or oscillating cast-cutting saws can be used to cut a window in the plastron. Radiographs are useful for planning to avoid the humeral and pectoral girdles. Typically cuts are through the abdominal and femoral scutes. If one bevels the cut so that the outer surface is larger than the inner (coloemic) surface, the plastron repair is easier.[12] A four-sided cut is made, being especially careful of the large paired parallel abdominal veins anteriorly and posteriorly just off midline. If these veins are inadvertently cut, they can be ligated.[12] Keep cutting surfaces cool by dripping sterile saline on them while cutting. Once fully through the plastron, pry up the plastron while detaching coelomic muscles from the periosteum (do not detach periosteum from bone). If possible, leave the periosteum intact on the posterior or pelvic side to form a hinge.[113] This may speed healing. Once the hinge is up, immediatly control any bleeders. Vessels will vasospasm quickly but could hemorrhage postoperatively if not controlled.[113] Flush or sponge out the bone fragments from drilling that are lying on muscle and the coelomic membrane. One can carefully incise the coelomic membrane from the anterior limit, at the pericardial sac, to the posterior limit, at the transverse abdominal vein. The transverse abdominal vein joins the two ventral abdominal veins just under the pelvis. If more exposure is required, it can be ligated. Be careful not to incise the bladder through the coelomic membrane. Chelonians have a thicker uterus or shell gland than squamates. This makes salpingotomy, egg removal, and repair of the salpinx practical. The coelomic membrane should be sutured and the shell defect repaired with 5-minute epoxy as previously discussed.

Endoparasites

Fecal examinations are recommended for all chelonians. Nematodes are prevalent among captive chelonians but are considered nonpathogenic.[114] However, treatment is recommended because of the potential for superinfection in captivity and the direct life cycle of some species. Fenbendazole (Panacur, Hoecht-Roussel, suspension 10% or granules 22.2%) at 25 to 100 mg/kg via stomach tube or on food is recommended at 2-week intervals until ova are no longer detected by fecal examination (typically two to four treatments). The British suggest that oxfendazole (Systemex, Mallinckrodt) at 65 mg/kg once via stomach tube is an efficacious wormer.[111,115–118] Ivermectin (Ivomec 1%, MSD AGVET) causes flaccid paresis, paralysis, and death in chelonians, even at low doses,[119] and should not be used in chelonians.[120] Nematodes often exploit snails and fish as intermediate hosts. Avoid feeding snails and freeze fish for 3 days to reduce parasite transmission in aquatic turtles.

In an 18-month study,[121] roughly a quarter of a mixed group of red-footed (*Geochelone carbonaria*) and leopard (*G. pardalis*) tortoises died from verminous enterocolitis. Viviparous nematodes (*Proatractis*), which complete their life cycle without leaving the host, and overcrowding were incriminated. Box turtles and aquatic turtles can have a variety of one and two host flukes. Fluke eggs are large and colored and sink on fecal flotation. They can be detected in direct smears or in the sediment of fecal flotations. Adult flukes may be found in the gastrointestinal and respiratory systems. Generally flukes are considered nonpathogenic, but this may simply reflect lack of study.[122] Spirorchid blood flukes are considered pathogenic.[122] Widespread disposition of fluke eggs can result in listlessness, anorexia, occlusion of blood vessels, ulcerative shell lesions, pneumonia, central nervous systemic signs, stupor, and death.[122] Praziquantel (Droncit Injectable, Haver/Diamond), at 8 mg/kg SC, q 14 days for two treatments, is the drug of choice for trematode as well as cestode infections.

Protozoan infections are possible in tortoises, especially under crowded conditions. *Entamoeba invadens* caused high mortality in a group of recently imported red-footed tortoises.[123] Necropsy findings included necrosis of the duodenal surface and thickening and edema of the duodenal wall, multifocal fibrinous plaques in the colon, and necrosis of the common bile duct, gallbladder, and liver. The amoebae seemed to spread to the liver via the common bile duct and from showering from the renal portal system.[123] Treatment with dimetridazole solution in the food dramatically decreased mortality.

Flagellated protozoans, such as *Trichomona* and *Hexamita* spp., can also cause problems in tortoises. Protozoans can normally be found in small numbers (fewer than 10 per 400x field) in direct smears of feces or colonic washes.[120] When present in large numbers (more than 10 per 400x field) they can cause acute anorexia, polydipsia, diarrhea, and passage of undigested food in the feces. Metronidazole is an effective treatment at 100 mg/kg q 14 days via stomach tube for two treatments.

Acanthocephalans, thorny-headed worms, are common in wild-caught aquatic turtles. These worms attach to the wall of the stomach and small intestine and can cause enteritis of varying severity.[122]

Parasites are prevalent among chelonians. Typically they do not cause problems unless husbandry is inadequate. Nonetheless, treatment is recommended to avoid potential problems. Fecal flotation will not detect flukes or protozoans. Examine the fecal flotation sediment for trematodes and direct smears of fresh feces or colonic or cloacal washes for protozoans.

Metabolic bone disease

This is a common disease of captive-raised chelonians, especially young growing animals.[94] If the turtle has developed a normal shell before the onset of metabolic bone disease (MBD), clinical signs may be difficult to appreciate. Dietary history often suggests MBD and nonspecific signs, such as lethargy and anorexia, are often present. In growing turtles, clinical signs are more apparent, especially with regard to the shell. Abnormal shell findings include a soft shell, perhaps with uneven surfaces or ventral convexities of the carapace, a shell that seems too small for the turtle, and dorsal curling of the carapace marginals (figure 20). Other signs of MBD include a curved anterior maxilla that resembles a parrot's beak (figure 20), increased vertical growth of the bridge area (figure 20), lack of growth or appetite, curving of the normally straight ventral or dorsal midline scutes, and appendicular fractures. Hatchling tortoises on a good diet should develop a firm shell in about a year.[94] Penile prolapse may be present (figure 19) and severe cases cannot lift their shell while ambulating. The author suspects subclinical metabolic bone disease in many cases of pyramidal shell growth (figure 21). Radiographs may reveal decreased opacity to appendicular pillars and increased netlike porosity to shell in mild cases, to obvious lack of bone density in severe cases. Treatment is similar to that for iguanas[94,107]; see metabolic bone disease in chapter 3.

Starvation

Starvation is often encountered in conjunction with hypovitaminosis A or inadequate husbandry. An underweight turtle feels light for its shell size (see weight evaluation earlier in this chapter) and is often dehydrated as well. For tortoises, one can compare the patient's weight to estimated body weight ($= 0.191 \times SCL^3$). The temporal muscles may be obviously atrophied and the eyes sunken in the orbits.

Treatment should focus on rehydration before nutrition. See the subsections on stomach tubing and fluid administration earlier in this chapter for more information. Tube feeding chelonians is generally a two-person procedure. It is easier to pass a tube down the esophagus with the neck extended. With the head and neck extended and the turtle held vertically, the maxilla is opened and a speculum inserted. Lubricate the tip of the feeding tube and pass it down the esophagus (avoid the glottis at the base of the tongue) to the center of the plastron where the stomach lies. Slight resistance is usually felt as the tube passes through the esophageal sphincter. Tube feed 20 ml/kg EOD of an avian hand-feeding formula slowly over a minute or so. Stop and remove the tube if the formula refluxes up the esophagus. Keep the neck extended and the turtle vertical for a minute after tube feeding.

Intestinal impaction

Sand, gravel, or other nondigestible material can slowly accumulate in the gastrointestinal tract of tortoises fed on these substrates. Keeping food off the substrate by using dishes or newspaper may avoid the problem altogether. Keep in mind that tortoises often consume small rocks and pebbles, and generally these pass without assistance. Symptoms of intestinal impaction or obstruction include anorexia, lethargy, dehydration, constipation, and obstipation. Radiographs often reveal accumulation of radiopaque foreign material, especially if it protrudes dorsally into the lung fields on the horizontal lateral view. Leukocytosis or leukopenia may be present and cloacal or inguinal palpation may be abnormal.[124] Initial treatment consists of epicoelomic rehydration, broad-spectrum antibiotics, repeated stomach tubing with petroleum-based laxatives dissolved in water, and mineral oil enemas every 2 to 3 days. Physillium husks are often used for sand colic in horses, due to their hydroscopic nature, and are also indicated for use in tortoises. Twice-daily soaking in shallow lukewarm water (27°C [80°F]) for half an hour may promote gastrointestinal peristalsis. If symptoms of metabolic bone disease or hypocalcemia are present, calcium supplementation is indicated. Most cases resolve within several weeks with persistent conservative treatment. Regurgitation is a poor prognostic indicator; consider celiotomy and enterotomy for long-term impactions or large foreign bodies.[124] Be forewarned that the short mesentery of the chelonian intestinal tract makes elevation of the intestines through the plastral celiotomy impossible. Accordingly, make the osteotomy site as large as feasible to allow one to work within the shell.[125] Inguinal celiotomy is not recommended for the same reason.

For Further Reading

One of the best books on chelonian husbandry is that by Highfield.[73] Other useful references for natural history and captive care include Boycott and Bourquin,[72] de Vosjoli,[75,126,127] Ernst and Barbour,[128] Highfield,[115] McArthur,[111] Pritchard,[129] and Swingland and Klemens.[130]

3

Green Iguanas

Introduction to Green Iguanas

The green iguana, *Iguana iguana*, is a large, diurnal, semiarboreal, sedentary folivore found from Mexico to Brazil. Most veterinary problems in iguanas are a direct result of poor husbandry. Thus it is incumbent upon the veterinarian to be a knowledgeable source of good husbandry for the owner.

Natural history

Iguana habitat is generally found within 50 m of water. Iguanas prefer to sleep on branches overhanging water. If disturbed at night, they drop into the water for escape. Iguanas bask for about 4 hours in the morning to raise their body temperature for foraging.[131] Once warm, they leave their tree for foraging on the ground and in nearby trees and shrubs. Studies in Panama found that iguanas ate leaves, fruit, and flowers of select herbs, shrubs, trees, and vines in short frequent feeding bursts concentrated from late morning to early afternoon.[132] Most plant species in the diet were abundant, but the lizards exerted effort to eat less common species and seasonally available foods. Although a wide variety of plant species were eaten, stomach contents typically consisted of one or two species, and researchers speculate that dietary diversity is accomplished over a period of days rather than daily.[132] Until recently, it was assumed that younger animals were partially insectivorous to facilitate rapid growth, but now it is believed that iguanas are herbivorous throughout life,[132,133] although they occasionally accept carrion, secondarily ingest insects, and cannibalize small iguanas.[134–136] Growing iguanas achieve faster growth rates by selecting diets higher in digestible protein (by selecting new growth on plants) and maintaining higher body temperatures, which is believed to increase digestive efficiency.[133] New growth also has a higher calcium content and it is likely that young growing iguanas select a diet that is richer in calcium than adults' diets. During midday iguanas are immobile the majority of their time, perhaps resting and conserving energy.[131] They typically bask for another 2 to 3 hours in the afternoon. Several hours before sunset they return to their sleeping trees and remain there until sunrise.[131]

Studies indicate that iguanas are not territorial except during breeding season.[131] Nonmating iguanas express only mild protests to being passed on a branch and quickly return to normal. However, they prefer to keep distance between one another and do not seek one another's company.

In Venezuela, breeding season begins in early November.[131] Males select sites within their home range that exhibit the largest concentration of females. Initially territorial defense is intermittent but as November wears on the males become increasingly aggressive. Males decrease foraging, lose weight, and begin regularly patrolling their territorial boundary. Male combat consists of short wrestling matches with biting of the extremities. Small individuals from both sexes are excluded from these territories except for nighttime roosting.

Once territories are established, male behavior falls into one of three types.[131] Pseudofemales are small adult males that do not display, head bob, or attempt to mate. Rodda[131] believes that other iguanas of both sexes mistake pseudofemales for females. Peripheral males are medium adult males that stay at the periphery of a territorial male's territory. Peripheral males sneak forced copulations on females by intercepting foraging females or by forays into the territorial male's territory. Territorial males are generally large iguanas that defend specific areas with females present.

Females become receptive to breeding in late November or early December. As their bodies fill with developing follicles, they cease foraging and remain in trees all day long. A female dominance hierarchy, based on size, develops within territories, perhaps in an attempt to keep nonresident females out of their male's territory.[131] Females may be mated by several males and switch territories. Males usually mate once per day. After breeding season, territorial males begin feeding as territorial patrolling and male aggression wane.

Green Iguana Care

Oviposition

Females eat less and less as the eggs develop. De Vosjoli[137] noted that normal captive females go off feed for 3 to 5 weeks prior to oviposition. Females in Panama lay clutches of 23 to 60 eggs (the mean is 40) from late January to mid-March during the dry season.[138] In Costa Rica and Mexico, eggs are laid in March and early April. Larger females lay larger clutches. Females in captivity tend to produce less eggs than their wild counterparts. Hatchlings appear in 90 days at the start of the rainy season. Under artificial incubation at 27 to 35°C (80.6 to 95°F) eggs hatch in approximately 93 days.[138]

Females nest solitarily or in groups and can travel several kilometers to reach nest sites.[139] In Panama, iguanas prefer to nest on small islands, beaches, and open savanna. Researchers have found complex burrow systems shared by multiple females that are reused annually. It is tempting to speculate that a lack of suitable nesting areas is one reason females often fail to lay in captivity. Werner and Miller[140] felt that the composition of nesting substrate was less important than just having something to dig down into.

In captivity, nest boxes can be constructed many ways. De Vosjoli[137] recommends a tall, rectangular, plastic, kitchen trash can, laid on its side and filled with 50% potting soil and 50% sand. A hole can be cut in the lid big enough for the iguana to crawl through. A large rectangular plastic storage box (roughly 2 x 2 x 3 feet long) also works well. Frye and Townsend[141] recommend a medium-sized doghouse with a removable lid and a 30-cm board nailed across the entrance. The inside can be filled with a mixture of slightly moistened sand and sphagnum moss. Alternatively, a cat litter box, filled with suitable substrate, can be enclosed within a cardboard box, with a small entrance cut at one end. Another simple design is a large-diameter clay or PVC pipe (15 to 20 cm wide and 100 cm long) with a removable seal at one end.[142] The closed half of the pipe can be filled with suitable substrate. Nest boxes should be placed in the warmest corner of the cage as soon as the female is sexually mature or exhibits signs of gravidity such as eating less, increasing abdominal size, restlessness, pacing, and digging. It is probably better to have the nest box present year-round.

Sexing

Mature iguanas are easy to sex because the ventral femoral pores are larger in males (figure 22). Mature males have hemipenal bulges at the ventral tail base, larger scales on the face and dorsal spinous crests, larger dewlaps and jowls, and grow much larger. In addition, males from Central America develop a bronze orange color dorsally with sexual maturity during the breeding season. Females can also become orange. These differences are not detectable in hatchlings and are subtle in juveniles. Smaller iguanas are easily probed, males probe much deeper than females (figure 23). Males typically probe caudolaterally a depth equal to the tail base dorsoventral height, females less than half this. Secondary sex characteristics become distinguishable at sexual maturity. Sexing from small amounts of blood is also commercially available from Zoogen Inc. (1756 Picasso Ave., Davis, CA 95616). Sexual maturity is typically achieved at 2 to 3 years (if growing normally) or once above 500 g. Breeding is usually not successful until the third year in captivity.

Housing

In captivity, iguanas grow rapidly (30 to 60 cm per year), reaching adult size within 2 to 3 years.[143,144,145] Iguanas can live 10 to 15 years if properly fed and cared for and perhaps twice this length in rare instances. Owners should invest in a larger aquarium initially or be prepared to purchase a large one later. A 20-gallon aquarium is adequate for juveniles, but within a few years most owners must build larger glass, plywood, and screen cages. Wood should be laminated or caulked and sealed with an undercoat of water sealant and two to three coats of nontoxic sealant, such as polyurethane (let the cage air out for a week before placing an animal in it). Melamine is another good option; seal the seams well or it will warp. Provide as much vertical space as practical to accommodate their arboreal lifestyle. Screened cages are ideal for partial sunlight exposure outdoors in warmer months.

Iguanas stay apart from one another in a natural habitat except for breeding. Ideally, one should house iguanas individually in captivity[144] or provide a large enough cage, such as a room, so that iguanas can space themselves. Unfortunately, this is generally impractical, and it is common for iguanas to be kept in groups. This often works for same-sized juveniles, but as size disparity emerges, problems develop. The larger iguana dominates food and heat sources. In turn, the smaller iguana fails to thrive and may suffer from chronic stress. As the size disparity increases, the larger iguana may actually attack or kill the smaller iguana (figure 24). Barten[146] mentions symptoms in the subordinate lizard of slow growth, emaciation, poor muscle tone, poor color, lethargy, and susceptibility to infections and parasites. It is best to house iguanas individually.

As adults, males are intolerant of other males and immature females. Males may tolerate the presence of a few mature females but stable groups are difficult to maintain. Males may kill females and females may fight among themselves.[147] Even iguanas that have been housed together for years may abruptly start fighting. Severe trauma can result. Several smaller cages are preferable to one large communal cage.

It is not advisable to allow iguanas free roam of the house because of the numerous hazards they can encounter.[143] Barten[143] notes that lizards allowed to roam free are subject to chilling because of lack of access to heat sources, drafts from under doors, and cold outer walls and windows. Dogs, ferrets, and cats particularly like to attack iguanas. Iguanas are also subject to trauma from being stepped on, closed in doors, and falling. They may also eat things that are not good for them, such as nails and tacks, and spread bacteria throughout the house (see *Salmonella* section in chapter 1).

Substrates

The bottom of the cage should be lined with newspaper (the cheapest and easiest to use), indoor–outdoor carpeting, medium to large wood chips (large enough that they cannot be eaten) mixed with peat moss and sphagnum moss, orchid bark, pine bark mulch, alfalfa pellets, sphagnum moss, potting soil, or earth. Avoid sand, gravel, kitty litter, crushed corncobs, or crushed walnut shells because they can cause numerous problems and are difficult to clean.[143,144] If potting soil is used, make sure to remove perlite, if present, or the iguana may selectively eat it. If indoor–outdoor carpeting is used, get a second carpet so that a clean, dry one can be substituted while the other is washed and dried. Watch for frayed edges, which iguanas like to ingest, which could develop into a string foreign body. If using newspaper or indoor–outdoor carpeting, cages should be cleaned weekly (or sooner if dirty). The others should be completely changed every several months, but feces and moldy alfalfa pellets need to be scooped out regularly. Constantly moist or filthy environments are potential sources of infection. Rinsing with hot water is enough for most cleanings; more thorough cleaning with a 5% bleach solution is warranted periodically.

Housing accessories

Hardwood driftwood branches for climbing and basking are appreciated. A water bowl big enough for the iguana to enter and soak in is also needed and should be cleaned whenever dirty or at least twice a week.

Frye and Townsend[141] stress that iguanas need access to water at all times, not just once a week. In the native state, iguanas are often found in close association with water.

Hatchling iguanas are very prone to retain shed skin on the toes and tail, perhaps as a result of low humidity in captivity. As retained shed skin builds up on toes or tails, it gradually compromises circulation and avascular necrosis may result. One way to avoid this is to provide a humid retreat in an otherwise dry cage. For example, a plastic shoe or sweater box can be filled halfway with damp vermiculite or sphagnum moss and an entrance cut into one side or the lid. One can boost humidity in drier parts of the country by spraying daily or using a humidifier. Retained shed skin on the toes and tail should be removed before it becomes a problem (see digital and tail necrosis later in this chapter).

Temperature

Iguanas spend much of their day in the tropics soaking up the sun and prefer warmer conditions than most reptiles. Studies of iguanas in a natural habitat found that they keep their body temperature well above ambient temperature. Active iguanas found at midday ambient temperatures of 27.8 to 32.2°C (82 to 90°F) had cloacal temperatures of 32.8 to 37.8°C (91 to 100°F). Sleeping iguanas found at ambient temperatures of 23.9 to 25.6°C (75 to 78°F) had cloacal temperatures of 23.9 to 27.2°C (75 to 81°F), respectively. Numerous studies of wild iguanas have shown that adult iguanas, by basking in the sun, maintain daytime body temperatures between 36 and 37°C (96.8 and 98.6°F). It is probably not coincidental that iguanas have body temperatures similar to those of mammalian hind gut fermenters.[133]

In captivity, the ideal cage temperature should not drop below 21.1°C (70°F) at night and gradually rise to between 29.4 and 32.2°C (85 and 90°F) during the day with a localized hot spot or basking area between 35 and 37.8°C (95 and 100°F). This will allow the iguana to regulate its own body temperature and ensure proper digestion of food through behavioral thermoregulation. Large iguanas can tolerate temperatures 5°F beyond the preceding ranges.

There are many ways to provide the aforementioned thermal gradients, but keep in mind that, because each setup is different, it is impossible to predict what works in each situation. Therefore it is essential that the owner monitor temperatures. Inexpensive indoor–outdoor, minimum–maximum, digital thermometers are widely available from electronics stores. The basking area can be provided by placing a 60- to 100-watt incandescent light bulb, with reflector, outside the cage or resting on the screen top so that it warms a branch or rock in the cage. Small glass or porcelain infrared lights also work well, but make sure they are at least 18 inches from the iguana (see temperature section in chapter 1). With either light, make sure the iguana cannot come into direct contact with or too close to the light, or serious thermal burns may result. Iguanas have been known to hang directly on light bulbs while their skin slowly burns!

The best way to heat the rest of the cage is with a space heater keeping the room between 24 and 32°C (75 and 90°F). Other less desirable heat sources include heat tape, heating pads, or hot rocks. Again, make sure heating sources hot enough to burn the iguana are not present within the cage without safeguards. Anything too hot to rest a hand on, or under, for several minutes, may eventually burn the reptile (figure 25). Heating sources outside the cage are much safer. If the iguana spends most of its time on a hot rock, this is an indication the ambient temperature is too cool.

Feeding

Captive diets for green iguanas are constantly being reevaluated as we learn more. Unfortunately, controlled studies are scarce; therefore most diets are empirical. It is important to keep an open mind, because current recommendations may change as more is learned. Commercial iguana diets offer an obvious convenience; unfortunately, some are nutritionally inadequate and the safety of others remains to be seen.[148] Until controlled studies are done it is safest to feed as wide a variety of foods as possible and not rely on any one food for the bulk of the diet.

In the past, protein-rich foods, such as mammalian chows, were recommended by many authors (including this one). This was based on the mistaken notion that young iguanas were partially insectivorous and the desire to combat an epidemic of metabolic bone disease. Times change and we now know that a varied vegetarian diet, with calcium supplementation and UV light, will allow normal growth in iguanas. Mammalian chows, insects, and rodents may actually be detrimental to iguanas. Barten[148] points out that other herbivores, such as cows or rabbits, grow well without supplementing them with dog food, and we should approach iguana nutrition with a similar mindset. Iguanas are primarily folivores (leaf eaters), so it makes sense to feed them a ration heavily dependent on dark leafy greens. Accordingly, iguana rations should include 95% vegetables and 5% fruits. A common misconception is that iguanas will select a balanced diet from the foods offered. Although this may be true in a natural habitat, it is certainly not true of captive iguanas. Foods listed in bold print have a positive calcium-to-phosphorus ratio and should provide the bulk of the diet.[147]

> **95% Vegetables**—The majority of the diet should consist of dark leafy greens. Dark leafy greens that are rich in calcium include **collard, mustard,** and **turnip tops** or **greens, kale, Chinese cabbages (bok choy, pak choi), broccoli rabe** or **rapina (leaves from the broccoli plant,** not the florets humans are fond of), **clover,** and **dandelions (flowers, stems, and leaves)**. Other dark leafy greens include red or green cabbages, **Swiss chard, beet greens, escarole, parsley, spinach, watercress,** savoy, and kohlrabi. Light leafy greens include most lettuces. Lettuces tend to be mineral poor compared with the greens listed in bold print but

are fine in moderation. Romaine lettuce is preferable to other lettuces and iguanas love it. Be careful the iguana does not start eating lettuces to the exclusion of other foods. Flowers such as **roses, nasturtiums, carnations, dandelions,** and **hibiscus** are excellent. **Mulberry** and **hibiscus leaves** are good if available. Backyard grasses and weeds can provide free forage. Note that the outer darker leaves of most vegetables have a higher mineral content then the inner lighter leaves. Other types of vegetables include alfalfa, radish, clover and bean sprouts, soaked alfalfa pellets, asparagus, bell peppers, Brussels sprouts, carrots, cauliflower, cucumbers, green beans, jicama, mushrooms, okra, shredded parsnips, peas and pea pods, spineless **prickly pear cactus pads** (shave off the spine stubble), shredded summer or winter squashes, sweet potatoes, and uncooked thawed frozen mixed vegetables (corn, green beans, lima beans, peas, carrots).

Several dietary misconceptions abound among iguana owners.[149] One is that members of the cabbage family (cabbage, kale, Brussels sprouts, etc.), being goitrogens, will cause thyroid deficiencies if fed. This would be a potential concern if fed exclusively, but as part of a balanced diet they are certainly nutritious and will cause no thyroid problems.[16] Another misconception is that oxalates found in spinach, beets, Swiss chard, peas, and cabbage will limit calcium absorption from the gastrointestinal tract. As part of a balanced diet, these foods are nutritious and will cause no problems. Wild iguanas often select foods with a high oxalate content.[133] The latest dietary misconception is that frozen mixed vegetables will cause thiamin deficiencies. Again, as part of a balanced diet, frozen vegetables are fine in moderation.

5% Fruits—Fruits, in general, are mineral poor yet tasty enough that iguanas will eat them preferentially over more nutritious foods. Therefore limit fruits to 5% or less of the total ration. **Figs** are one of the few fruits rich in calcium.

> Apples, apricots, dates, **grapes,** kiwis, melons, mangos, peaches, **papayas,** pears, plums, prunes, raisins, star fruit, strawberries, tomatoes, and **raspberries** are all fine in small amounts. Iguanas are fond of bananas, unfortunately, banana is rich in phosphorus and calcium poor and should be fed sparingly.

To make a salad, wash, chop, and mix two or more types of dark leafy greens, several types of fresh or frozen vegetables, sprouts, and one to two fruits. Be careful to remove and discard any wires or rubber bands. It is better to chop up the salad by hand. Food processors tend to turn the salad into mush, which reduces roughage and speeds spoilage. If hand chopped, the vegetable portion can be stored for a week in the refrigerator but must be allowed to come to room temperature for an hour or so before feeding. Fruit can be added as a top-dressing just before feeding. For hatchlings, it is important to chop food into smaller pieces. Each week vary the diet by offering different foods.

Variety is the key to a healthy diet! All of the items mentioned can be found in grocery stores and should be fed. Until more is known, it is prudent not to rely on any one item for the majority of the diet. Most cases of metabolic bone disease presented to the author have had less than 5 to 10 different foods in the entire diet. It is important that the iguana eats what is offered and not just select foods; mixing the salad well should ensure this. Established bad dietary habits can take months to correct, and correction is crucial for long-term survival. Finicky eaters can be encouraged to eat more by mixing preferred foods in heavily at first and then gradually decreasing them over a few weeks. Be more stubborn than the iguana.

How much to feed is a tricky question. In general, feed enough that the lizard continues to gain weight and grow but not so much that it becomes obese. If the iguana eats all the food offered and still seems hungry, feed it more. Iguanas are best fed daily, especially hatchlings.

After roughly 6 months, they can be fed a minimum of three times per week or every other day. Daily feeding is more laborious but probably much better.

Calcium and multivitamin supplementation

Every feeding, sprinkle a light dusting of calcium carbonate, citrate, lactate, or gluconate on the salad. Do not oversupplement with calcium! A fine, barely perceptible dusting is all that is required. Phosphorus- and vitamin D-free calcium sources are recommended for regular usage, as vegetables tend to contain excess phosphorus and too much vitamin D is a potential concern. Multivitamins do not contain enough calcium to prevent metabolic bone disease (regardless of what the label implies). If the iguana will not eat the salad dusted with calcium, too much calcium is being added. A little less can be added, or the salad can be tossed more, but do not omit the calcium or metabolic bone disease will inevitably occur. Substitute a light dusting of good-quality multivitamins for the calcium no more than once or twice a month. Regular ultraviolet light exposure, with either natural sunlight or artificial fluorescent light, permits good bone growth (see ultraviolet light section in chapter 1).

Acclimatization

Wild-caught iguanas are often shy and should be minimally disturbed until they are eating well and seem less nervous. Have owners resist the temptation to try to tame them immediately, because it might be too much for an animal that is already maximally stressed. Allow them a few months to adjust to captivity and start feeding well. A hide box will give them a secure area in the cage for retreat. Particularly nervous individuals may need the cage covered so that they do not bash their snouts whenever there is movement outside the cage or pace constantly along the glass barrier.

Basic Medical Techniques for Green Iguanas

Restraint and handling

Several simple tricks make iguanas much easier to work with. Iguanas are easily startled by rapid movements from above, perhaps because arboreal raptors are one of their primary predators. Moving slowly around iguanas makes them much less likely to try to flee. Nail trims prior to handling cut down on scratches of the handler and can generally be accomplished without restraint. Use dog toenail trimmers for large iguanas and scissors or fingernail trimmers for smaller iguanas. Iguanas typically initially object to foot manipulation but calm down, after several attempts, if one persists and moves slowly. An elevated stool provides a suitable perch for an iguana, which it is usually content to stay on if no higher areas to climb up to are accessible. Iguanas struggle minimally if supported from below, such as stretched out on a forearm or upper thigh, if they are not disturbed.

For physical examination more secure restraint is needed. If the iguana is held from below or grabbed by the neck behind the head from above (as is typical in lizard restraint), the needle-sharp nails of the iguana will quickly shred the restrainer enough to make a mean cat look mild. A better approach (i.e., scratchless) is to first grab the pelvis, from above, placing a thumb and forefinger anterior to the rear legs, with the second finger behind. Iguanas may try to but typically cannot bite a hand with a firm grip on the pelvis. The iguana may struggle initially, but if you hold on, the head can quickly be restrained with the other hand. This is best done on a flat surface, so that if the iguana tries to roll, it can be pinned against the surface. Once it is calm, you can pick up the iguana, but quickly get it away from anything it can smack its tail against. The rear limbs can be placed between your thighs, taped to the tail, or wrapped in a towel to free the caudal hand for physical examination. Obviously, one should not handle suspected gravid or metabolic bone disease cases in this way!

Remember, iguanas will shed their tail if physically restrained by it while struggling to escape; this is particularly true of smaller lizards that are grabbed distally. Most larger iguanas can be gently manipulated by the base of the tail or even lifted for short periods if they do not struggle vigorously.

Physical examination

Before physical examination, obtain a good husbandry and medical history. Observe the lizard walking; normal iguanas lift their trunk and proximal tail well up off the ground, no matter how smooth the surface. Iguanas with metabolic bone disease (MBD) are often unable to lift some or all of their trunk up off the ground or may be limping. Gravid iguanas have distended caudal coeloms. Those with either condition should be handled with extreme caution or perhaps not at all. Iguanas with MBD are prone to fracture and spinal injury, and gravid females may rupture eggs, follicles, or the oviduct. After assessment of the likelihood of either condition, physical examination can proceed.

Physical examination is a matter of personal preference. Method is not as important as developing a routine and sticking to it every time. The author first restrains the iguana, then starts at the head. Grasp the head with a thumb and forefinger placed laterally, just behind the head, caudal to the commissures of the jaws. The free hand, from the pelvis, can tap the snout several times. Often the lizard will open its mouth enough for a quick oral examination. If not, occlude both nares with your fingers or tap the snout a little more annoyingly. If the lizard will not open its mouth, move the hand forward from the back of the head to restrain the upper mandible. With your other hand, apply steady downward traction to the dewlap and the mouth will open. You will need an assistant to restrain larger lizards. Use oral specula sparingly as they tend to damage the teeth, even if flexible. The teeth will regrow, but it is understandably disconcerting to the owner, not to mention the patient. Do not pry open the mouth or gingival damage will result. Iguanas are capable of severe bites, so be careful. Examine the oral cavity for abscesses, pallor, glottal discharge, lacerations, foreign bodies, or anything abnormal. Iguanas have a large fleshy tongue with a reddened split tip. The oropharynx is best observed with bright light. Pushing craniodorsally on the throat forces the glottis up into better view. Iguanas excrete salt through their nares, which can be seen as white deposits around the nares or deposited on glass in the cage. Owners are often under the misapprehension that this indicates a respiratory tract infection. Palpate the skull and all limbs, anterior to pelvis (for kidney enlargement), and as much of the coelom as feasible. Examine the vent, tail base, and toes. With major gastrointestinal disease, coelomic palpation may be painful; the iguana may arch its back, or regurgitate, or bloating may be present. In large iguanas, the kidneys can be palpated rectally if needed. The key to a good physical examination is to move slowly and palpate gently; rapid movements tend to alarm iguanas. Complete the physical examination with an accurate weight (always!) and sex determination (see sexing in previous section).

Phlebotomy

Bleeding iguanas is relatively easy compared with other reptiles. The caudal tail vein is the preferred site and can be bled with a 20- to 25-gauge heparinized needle long enough to reach the center of the tail. To avoid the hemipenes in male lizards, select a ventral midline site, one-fourth to one-third of the tail length down from the cloaca. Disinfect the venipuncture site, and insert the needle at a 45- to 60-degree angle to the posterior surface of the tail, until contact with the ventral vertebral body, where the caudal tail vein courses. Be aware that iguanids have large chevrons, which are ventral vertebral spinous processes, that course caudally from the vertebral body at a 45-degree angle. If resistance is encountered while inserting the needle, reinsert the needle, anteriorly or posteriorly, to avoid the chevron. Apply gentle plunger pressure until blood appears in the hub; some redirection is often needed. It is important to stay precisely on midline; palpate the dorsal spines for orientation. If no blood appears after several attempts, the needle could be clogged. Larger iguanas are easily bled by a single person, by allowing the iguana to hang vertically, on the inside of a cage door, from the horizontal struts. Restrain the tail base with one hand and bleed with the other. The tail vein can also be bled with the iguana's tail hanging off a table. The large ventral midline abdominal vein is not recommended, because of difficulty with hemostasis and the large potential space for hemorrhage.

Reptiles generally have blood volumes of 5% to 8% of their mass. Assuming one can collect 10% of a reptile's blood volume without harm, it would be safe to collect 0.5 to 0.8 ml of blood from a 100-g juvenile.[150] Serum separators are useful for biochemical profiles with limited amounts of blood. One can run a full chemistry panel with as little as 0.3 ml of whole blood (because of the relatively low PCV) and a complete blood count with 0.2 ml of blood.

Radiography

Radiographic technique is similar to the standard small-animal tabletop technique. Radiographic examination should include a dorsal ventral view with the iguana resting directly on the rare earth plate. Patiently position the iguana symmetrically, with slow movement and no distraction; the iguana will generally hold still. Placing a small towel over the head is often helpful. Lawton[151] recommends using a blinker system by placing a wad of cotton over each eye and wrapping over the eyes and around the head with self-adhesive bandage. The light pressure on the eyes through the eyelids induces the vagovagal response, which seems to relax the patient as heart rate slows. The lateral radiograph should be in a repeatable position to be most useful. Trying to restrain an iguana manually in lateral recumbency is frustrating, needlessly exposes the radiographer to radiation, and often results in overshadowing of the coelom with the limbs. An easier technique is to tape the wrists or forearms together and the femurs and knees to the tail base (figure 26). The iguana is then placed in lateral recumbency with one hand holding the tail and the other hand stretching the wrists anteriorly, with a large wooden spoon or stick. This technique not only results in good lateral alignment but also pulls all limbs out of the coelomic picture (figure 27). Strangely enough, in such bondage, iguanas seem more calm and struggle minimally. A more difficult alternative is the horizontal beam radiograph, with the lizard perched on foam and its front and rear legs drawn out of the coelomic picture. Dental radiographs are useful for appendicular pictures of small lizards and foot pictures of large lizards.

Fluid and injection sites

Although intravenous fluid administration is possible in iguanas, enteral, subcutaneous, or intracoelomic fluids are more practical. Fortunately, even very dehydrated iguanas absorb fluids well. Maintenance fluid volumes are estimated to be between 15 (large animals) and 25 (small animals) ml/kg/day administered in one or two doses.[12] For severe dehydration one can administer up to 40 ml/kg/day divided q 12 hr. An equal mixture of 5% dextrose or 0.45% NaCl added to nonlactated crystalloids are recommended;[90] however, other crystalloid fluids have been used successfully.[152] See subsection on fluid administration in Basic Medical Techniques for Turtles, Tortoises, and Terrapins in chapter 2 for more information. Take care to avoid lung and air sac areas (i.e., anteriodorsal two-thirds of coelom) at all times, because it is exceedingly easy to slip inadvertently through the ribs into the lungs. Subcutaneous fluids can be given in either the caudolateral body wall, the lateral tail base, or dorsal or caudal to the femurs. Intracoelomic fluids are given in the extreme caudal coelom, craniodorsal to femur and ventral to lumbar musculature.

Twenty- to 22-gauge needles are easily placed in the proximal, medial, tibial crest of larger iguanas[153] for intraosseous fluid administration and are well tolerated (figure 28). Sterile technique and local or general anesthesia are needed. This is an excellent method for continuous fluid administration with a fluid pump.

Antibiotics can be delivered orally through a syringe case past the tongue (see the following section on stomach tubing). As with most animals, once the pill is past the tongue it is generally swallowed. It is uncertain how well iguanas digest coated pills, so it may be well to crush pills, or empty capsules into water, before administration. Antibiotics can be injected in the muscle masses of the front legs or neck. Once again, avoid injecting over the lung areas.

Stomach tubing

Peroral fluids are an option if the patient is alert and vigorous. A stomach tube should be utilized to avoid aspiration. Stomach volume is estimated to be 1.5% (large iguana) to 2.5% (small iguana) of body weight or 15 to 25 ml/kg. Every-other-day feeding is recommended with fluids given via stomach tube on alternate days. Stomach tubes should be passed to the cranial third of the distance between front and rear legs. For small iguanas (< 200 g) small ball-tipped gavage tubes, tuberculin, or 0.3-cc Becton Dickinson insulin syringes (with needle removed), intravenous (IV) tubing, or red rubber catheters, cut to size, all work well for stomach tubing. For larger iguanas, a mouth speculum is needed to pass a stomach tube. A 1- to 3-cc syringe case, with both ends open, makes an effective, inexpensive, disposable speculum. To place a syringe case as a speculum, one person must hold open the mouth with steady traction on the mandibles and dewlap. A second person then places the open-ended syringe case straight back into the center of the mouth, as far posteriorly as possible. As the iguana bites down the first person can adjust the grip to hold the mouth shut on the speculum (figure 29). A stomach tube can then be easily passed down the center of the syringe case. This technique rarely results in tooth damage and is easily accomplished by owners at home. Larger lizards can be stomach tubed with one part alfalfa pellets or powder, blended for several minutes, with two to four parts water. The alfalfa gruel should be given through a catheter tip syringe and a large bore (18 French) red rubber feeding tube. Emeraid II (LaFaber's, Odell IL) has been used for smaller iguanas by the author for years, with apparent good results. See Donoghue and Langenberg[154] for an in-depth discussion of nutritional support in reptiles.

Diseases of Green Iguanas

Metabolic bone disease*

The most common problem of captive green iguanas is metabolic bone disease (MBD), also referred to as nutritional secondary hyperparathyroidism, rickets, osteoporosis, osteomalacia, chronic calcium deficiency, fibrous osteodystrophy, or hypocalcemia. Metabolic bone disease is the result of insufficient dietary calcium, excessive dietary phosphorus, lack of vitamin D, or rarely primary kidney, liver, or parathyroid disease. This is primarily a disease of young growing animals. Once adult size is reached, with normal bone formation, MBD is much less common but still possible.

Two distinct forms of MBD are present.[156] The first, prevalent in growing lizards, is classic MBD, with symptoms referable to the skeletal system, such as fibrous osteodystrophy and fractures. The second, prevalent in adult iguanas, has symptoms secondary to hypocalcemia, such as paresis, tremors, or seizures. MBD affects all patients differently. Therefore, the clinician should be alert for any or all of the following signs as an indication of MBD.

> **Classic MBD**—In iguanas, the earliest consistent symptom of MBD is partial to complete lack of truncal lifting.[1] Normal iguanas lift their trunk and proximal tail up off the ground while walking, no matter how smooth the surface (figure 30). Early in MBD, iguanas lift the front half of the body, but drag the pelvis and tail along the ground (figure 31). As MBD becomes more advanced, iguanas cannot lift any of their body and eventually cannot move, even though their legs scramble furiously.

* This section revised with permission from Boyer.[155]

Another frequent finding is a pliable mandible and/or maxillae. In advanced cases, constant posterior traction from lower jaw musculature pulls the symphysis posteriorly and the mandible bows laterally, an underbite develops.[12] This is often exaggerated by fibrous osteodystrophy. Juvenile iguanas retain the rounded infantile skull shape. In rapidly growing iguanas, lack of weight gain can be an early warning sign of MBD, as can declining appetite, anorexia, or bloating. Juvenile iguanas should gain 5 to 10 g per week if properly fed.

Lameness, or reluctance to move, results from long-bone fractures or muscular weakness (figure 32). Fractures, even without a history of trauma, should arouse suspicion of MBD. Fractures of the distal radius and ulna may create a false joint, proximal to the wrist, shifting weight bearing from the foot to the forearm. Fibrous osteodystrophy is common in long bones, often associated with fracture. Fibrous osteodystrophy results from supportive fibrous tissue being laid down around calcium-deficient softened bone in an attempt to reinforce it. Superficially the limbs appear well fleshed but feel more like bone than flesh.[12]

Kyphosis, scoliosis, lordosis, or rear limb paresis (less commonly paralysis) can also develop, sometimes with a history of trauma, such as being dropped. Rear limb paresis has a guarded prognosis, as fecal or urinary incontinence may also be present.

Radiographs are not essential for diagnosis but confirm suspicion of MBD and are useful to assess fractures, etiology, and response to treatment. Radiographically there is an overall decrease in bone density (figure 33 versus figure 34). Poor bone contrast from soft tissue is especially noticeable in the pelvis, transverse processes of the caudal tail vertebrae (figure 33 versus figure 34), and dorsal spinous processes of vertebrae.[155] The cortices of long bones may have a dramatically widened outer cortex, with fibrous osteodystrophy (figure 33), or appear thinner than normal.[12] The medullary cavity is typically normal. Transverse folding fractures of the long bones and compression fractures of the vertebrae are common.[12]

Plasma calcium (Ca) and phosphorus (P) levels can be normal or there may be decreased Ca levels (< 9.5 mg/dl) and increased P levels (> 7.0 mg/dl). A negative Ca/P ratio is strong evidence of MBD. Unfortunately, normal Ca and P levels do not rule out MBD; in these cases, the clinician must carefully evaluate dietary history, any mild clinical signs, and radiographs.

Hypocalcemic MBD—This less common form is most often seen in adult iguanas. Intermittent muscle tremors are seen in the digits, limbs, or large muscle masses. Tremors become progressively more frequent and severe, especially with activity. Eventually seizures, tetany, or flaccid paresis develops. Generally these animals are hypocalcemic but, because of calcium homeostasis, not all animals are hypocalcemic at the time of sampling (especially if not currently symptomatic). In addition to the normal causes of MBD, a wide variety of conditions can cause similar symptoms, including thiamine, vitamin E, or selenium deficiency; septicemia; trauma; renal or hepatic disease; neoplasia; heavy parasite burdens; epilepsy; egg development; and insecticide or heavy metal toxicity, such as from zinc from pennies.[155,157] In the author's experience, frequent causes in adult iguanas include poor diet, renal failure, and oogenesis. Thorough diagnostic work-up, including a detailed dietary history, physical examination, plasma chemistry panel, complete blood count, radiographs, and fecal examination, is indicated.

Treatment—Before commencing treatment, it is imperative that the veterinarian discuss correction of all deficient aspects of husbandry with the owner. All the medicine in the world will not correct MBD if husbandry, especially the diet, is not improved. Most MBD cases are treated on an outpatient basis, with the exception of hypocalcemic patients. To avoid further fractures, handling should be minimized and climbing areas and cagemates removed. Natural sunlight or artificial sources of ultraviolet light and written instructions on proper diet are recommended. With follow-up examinations, if the patient is not eating enough to maintain or increase body weight, recovery from MBD will be prolonged. Tube feeding is indicated (see stomach tubing section in this chapter). Once the patient starts to grow and repair bone, recovery from MBD accelerates. If the patient is vigorous and not prone to aspiration, begin oral calcium supplementation with 1 ml/kg calcium glubionate (Neo-calglucon Syrup, USP) q 12 hr.[158] If the patient is suffering from hypocalcemic MBD and is not alert enough for oral supplementation, give 100 mg/kg 10% calcium gluconate (100 mg Ca/ml) intracoelomically q 6 hr or as needed to prevent muscle tremors. For iguanas, intracoelomic injections should be given dorsolaterally in the extreme caudal abdomen, just anterior to the pelvic limbs, rather than flipping over a struggling iguana for ventral injections. Begin oral calcium glubionate once the patient is stable and alert. Calcium glubionate should be continued until the patient is gaining weight and consuming calcium supplements on food, typically for 1 to 3 months. Calcium carbonate should be sprinkled, or dusted, on salads once the patient is feeding well and as calcium glubionate is tapered off. Balanced Ca-to-P supplements (such as bone meal) are no longer recommended for treatment of MBD because many of these patients are hyperphosphatemic.

Vitamin D (1000 IU/kg vitamin D, Injacom 100, Roche Animal Health and Nutrition) and Calcitonin (50 IU/kg calcitonin, Miacalcin, Schering Plough) injections are also recommended IM q 7 days for two treatments (longer if needed for calcitonin). Vitamin D is indicated only if dietary history suggests a lack thereof. If the patient is hypocalcemic (< 8.5 mg/dl) or the calcium status is unknown, do not give calcitonin until the patient is normocalcemic or allow several days of calcium glubionate therapy first.[158] Calcitonin is believed to speed recovery from MBD because it inhibits Ca resorption from bone and may negatively feed back and decrease parathyroid hormone secretion.

Fracture management—Appendicular fractures are best managed conservatively. For small patients with multiple fractures, cage rest is advisable. The benefits of fracture stabilization must be considered versus stress to the patient. The bones are too soft for surgical fixation. A variety of external coaptation methods work well including reinforced tape, Hexalite (Hexcel Medical Products), or Sam Splints (Jorgensen Labs).[157] Proximal femoral or multiple rear limb fractures are splinted dorsally over the pelvis.[148] Distal appendicular fractures are easily managed and well tolerated by taping the leg under traction to the posterior body wall, tail, or syringe case splint. See Bennett[159] for a review of fracture management. Perfect alignment is not required for good functional recovery.

Prognosis—With early detection, aggressive treatment, and good owner compliance, the prognosis is excellent. Without aggressive treatment, most symptomatic cases do not survive. Mild fibrous osteodystrophy disappears in time; severe fibrous osteodystrophy can be permanent. Scoliosis can become more problematic as the animal grows. Rear limb paralysis and fecal or urinary incontinence, secondary to compression fractures involving the spinal cord, have a poor prognosis. The hypocalcemic form of MBD has a more guarded prognosis, often dependent on the underlying cause. In general, classic MBD remains a reversible disease with a good prognosis, provided veterinary intervention and good owner compliance are obtained.

Renal failure

Renal failure is a frequent cause of death in older iguanas and is often associated with heavy feeding of mammalian chows and multivitamins. The etiology remains unknown. Frye[12,16] suspects that dog, cat, or monkey chow contributes too much vitamin D if it is more than 5% of the total diet. History often reveals long-term multivitamin supplementation several times per week. Owners often do not distinguish multivitamins from calcium supplements as most multivitamins contain calcium. Good dietary history will distinguish the two. Unfortunately, the same dietary history may apply to many healthy iguanas, making a cause-and-effect scenario difficult to prove. Lack of UV light, dehydration, suboptimal temperature, and excess dietary protein, fat, or phosphorus could also contribute to kidney failure.

Clinical signs of kidney failure are nonspecific, such as anorexia, weight loss, lethargy, flaccid paresis, or bloating. Hypocalcemic muscle tremors of the digits or appendicular muscles are much more suggestive but not always present. However, muscle tremors are often present in metabolic bone disease as well. Sometimes one can palpate enlarged kidneys anterior to the pelvis (figure 35) or in the dorsal cloaca. Normal iguana kidneys are sheltered within the pelvic inlet. As kidneys enlarge they occlude the caudal colon and distend beyond the pelvic inlet into the caudal coelom. Massive renomegaly may result in cloacal prolapse, obstipation, dyschezia, or coelomic pain or distention. Owners typically do not notice any changes associated with this. Sometimes the iguana urinates normally but has difficulty defecating, or the feces may be subtly elongated and tapered (figure 36). Iguanas may defecate only while soaking (which is not abnormal by itself) or defecate less frequently. In severe cases, intrapelvic kidney enlargement occludes the colon and prevents defecation.

Diagnosis of kidney failure can be frustrating. Most iguanas are minimally symptomatic until late in renal failure. Many iguanas are too small to palpate the kidneys cloacally. Poor contrast in the caudal abdomen hampers radiographic detection of kidney enlargement. Radiographs may reveal increased density of large blood vessels, especially noticeable in the lung fields. Sonagraphy would be ideal for detection of renal enlargement but is not currently utilized extensively. Lack of known normal kidney measurements and interference from the bony pelvis further limit use of ultrasound.

Reptiles do not concentrate their urine; thus urine specific gravity is not useful in early detection of renal disease. As iguanas are uricotelic, blood urea nitrogen and creatinine are only minimally elevated or normal. As with mammals and birds, uric acid and phosphorus become elevated late in kidney disease. In iguanas uric acid elevations are not as dramatic as in birds or other reptiles in renal failure. The mean plasma uric acid levels of a dozen iguanas with kidney failure[160] was 7.2 mg/dl with a standard deviation (SD) of 5.7 mg/dl, compared with normal ranges for 10 iguanas of 1.5 mg/dl with an SD of 0.4.[331] This may be because most iguanas in renal failure have not eaten recently and thus are not producing uric acid, or perhaps it is related to the lesional level of renal disease. Phosphorus is often dramatically elevated (two or four times normal) late in renal failure, yet other common problems, such as MBD and intestinal disease, can also cause elevations of phosphorus. Preliminary evidence[160] indicates that creatine, the metabolic precursor of creatinine, may offer another indicator of renal disease, but much work still needs to be done to prove this. However, creatine testing is not widely available at this time. Plasma chemistries suggestive of renal failure[160] include elevations of plasma phosphorus, creatine (not creatinine), and potassium and normal to decreased calcium. Uric acid may or may not be elevated.

Plasma aspartate aminotransferase (AST, SGOT), alanine aminotransferase (ALT, SGPT), alkaline phosphatase, and creatinine kinase (CK, CPK) are typically elevated, the last often dramatically. Leukocytosis with heterophilia is often present. If the animal is dehydrated, the PCV may be elevated.

On necropsy, pulmonary, mesenteric, and great vessels have a firm gritty consistency with a thickened lumen. The kidneys are often massively enlarged (figure 37). Microscopically one observes extraskeletal calcification in a wide array of tissues including heart, muscle, lung, renal tubules, and the central nervous system. Calcification of the tunica media is present in many vessels and there are nephrosis and interstitial fibrosis. Parathyroid hyperplasia may result in osteopenia with increased bone remodeling. If the patient has been anorexic, hepatic lipidosis may be present.

The prognosis for renal failure is grave to poor, as iguanas generally present in end-stage renal failure. If detected earlier, treatment could prolong life span and perhaps even reverse symptoms in borderline cases. Biopsies could be useful prognostically in such cases. If owners elect, treatment consists of curtailment of multivitamins and mammalian chows, diuresis with physiological saline at 20 to 30 ml/kg q 24 hr, and correction of fluid deficits over several days. Fluids may be given through intraosseous or intravenous catheters with a fluid pump or a combination of subcutaneous, intracoelomic, and enteral fluids, divided into several daily treatments. Watch for signs of overhydration, such as ocular discharge. Jarchow[161] suspects that iguanas in renal failure may be hypertensive. This seems a reasonable assumption given the widespread mineralization of the tunica media in blood vessels and the fact that many mammals in chronic renal failure are also hypertensive. If this is true, judicious use fluids and of antihypertensive agents may be beneficial.[161]

Barten[146] stresses that hypocalcemia must be treated with caution. In mammals, metastatic calcification is enhanced when the calcium phosphorus solubility product (SP) exceeds 70 mg/ml (SP = calcium mg/ml x phosphorus mg/ml). In mammals with renal compromise, the SP threshold decreases to 50 or 60 mg/ml. If the SP is less than 60 mg/ml, then calcium can be used to control muscle tremors. Give 100 mg/kg 10% calcium gluconate intracoelomically q 6 hr until the lizard is stable enough for oral supplements. Oral calcium glubionate is then given at 1 ml/kg q 12 hr. If the SP is greater than 60 mg/ml (which is typically the situation), additional calcium administration might promote further extraskeletal calcification. Diuresis may decrease the phosphorus level enough to supplement calcium, but it may also decrease the calcium level even further, inducing life-threatening hypocalcemia. In any case, serial plasma chemistry panels are important to evaluate therapy and monitor response to treatment.

Nutritional support with a phosphorus-restricted diet is also indicated but difficult as many vegetables are high in phosphorus. Fruits should be avoided altogether. As phosphorus restriction is generally inadequate to prevent hyperphosphatemia, phosphorus binding agents are also indicated. In treatment of human renal failure it is now thought that aluminum-containing drugs pose a risk for development of aluminum intoxication as aluminum is excreted through the kidneys.[162,163] The trend is to avoid use of aluminum products[163] or use them initially and replace them with calcium products once phosphorus is reduced to normal.[162] Calcium acetate, carbonate, and glubionate are currently in use as safer phosphorus binders.

Once again the prognosis, depending on the severity of clinical signs, is poor to guarded. In the author's experience, most patients with advanced renal failure fail to respond to treatment and are eventually euthanized or die early in treatment.

Cystic calculi

Cystic calculi can reach incredible sizes. The primary differential for a laminated radiopaque mass anywhere in the coelom of the iguana should be a bladder stone (figure 38); some can be surprisingly anterior. After removal by cystotomy, aggressive fluid therapy and good nursing care are important, but kidney damage is possible. Kidney failure is often associated with large uroliths, not because of urinary obstruction (the ureters empty into the cloaca, not the bladder) but perhaps because a diet producing excess uric acid may also predispose the iguana to gout. The diet should be corrected to limit uric acid precursors, such as purines. Foods known to be high in purines should be avoided. This includes most mammalian chows, rodents, and other foods such as asparagus, mushrooms, organ meat, anchovies, and sardines.

Neonatal iguanas

Hatchling green iguanas average 10 to 11 g and are fragile in inexperienced hands. They should be handled minimally until well established. If underweight (weight less than 10 g, legs and posterior abdomen not filled out, bony pelvic girdle), begin stomach tubing with avian hand-feeding formula every other day using a 0.3- to 1-cc syringe, starting with 0.1 ml and then increasing to 0.3 ml within 4 days. On alternate days, stomach-tube water instead. Correct husbandry and allow for behavioral thermoregulation up to 38°C (100°F).

Respiratory problems

Respiratory problems are rare in iguanas, except for hatchlings after being chilled. Clinical signs include increased respiratory effort, open-mouthed breathing, increased mucus in the oropharynx or discharging from the glottis, and decreased appetite. A normal hatchling iguana should be bright, alert, and responsive. Sick hatchlings keep their eyes closed except for brief periods of disturbance. Good nutritional support with stomach tubing, a warm environment, and injectable antibiotics for 3 to 6 weeks are indicated. Consider cytology and bacterial culture and sensitivity of glottal exudate or fluid from a tracheal wash. Remember that iguanas excrete salt through their nares and periodically sneeze salt. Owners occasionally observe this, especially on glass surfaces, and mistakenly interpret this as a sign of a respiratory tract infection. Iguanas in renal failure may hemorrhage through mineralized vessels anywhere in the body; if in the lungs, they may present with hemorrhagic glottal discharge.

Bloat

Neonatal bloat is an uncommon idiopathic problem (figure 39). In neonates bloat may present as an agonal problem in malnourished iguanas or as a complication of spinal injury secondary to metabolic bone disease[164] or perhaps secondary to hypocalcemia. Treatment has been largely unsuccessful but enemas, calcium supplementation, and antibiotics have saved rare cases. On necropsy the gastrointestinal tract is grossly distended with gas, often either the stomach and intestines or the cecum. No obstructions have been found.

In older iguanas bloat is often a symptom of other disease such as foreign bodies, obstructions, intussusceptions (especially iliocecal), and small intestinal or cecal volvulus. Symptoms are typical for coelomic distress, including pain with palpation, arching of the back, vomiting or regurgitation, and coelomic distention. Radiographs are often diagnostic (figure 27); coelomic exploration should proceed without delay. In the author's experience, vomiting or regurgitation is a serious symptom of major gastrointestinal disease in iguanas.

Exposure gingivitis

Previous MBD may slightly deform the mandible or maxillae and expose a small area of gingiva. The exposed oral mucosa is susceptible to exposure gingivitis but is not generally infected (figure 40). Frequent gentle cleaning with a Q-tip and application of lip balm generally control this problem. Owners are often under the mistaken notion this represents mouth rot.

Infectious stomatitis

Infectious stomatitis is rare in iguanas. It is often misdiagnosed when the normal reddish tongue tip is noted or exposure gingivitis is present. Symptoms of infectious stomatitis include gingival or pharyngeal inflammation, caseous exudate along the teeth, hypersalivation, and anorexia. Treatment consists of gently removing all cellular debris, cytology and culture with antibiotic sensitivities, systemic antibiotics, and supportive care if the iguana is malnourished. See infectious stomatitis in the section on snake diseases in chapter 5 for more information.

Abscesses and granulomas

Abscesses and granulomas are common on the head (especially along the posterior lateral mandible and rostrum; figure 41) and toes. Often these are mistaken for tumors that are uncommon in iguanas. Thoroughly examine the oral cavity with abscesses involving the head and do not overlook developing abscesses. Treatment includes surgical débridement under anesthesia, thorough flushing with dilute tamed iodine or chlorhexidine, and topical and systemic antibiotics. Consider aerobic and anaerobic cultures with sensitivities. Even severe abscesses respond well to treatment. For iguanas that continually run headlong into glass, tape paper over the glass.

Epidermal inclusion cysts

Epidermal inclusion cysts, analogous to canine sebaceous cysts, can be misdiagnosed as abscesses (because of secondary bacterial infections) and usually are on the dorsal or lateral tail (figure 42) or mandible. Treatment consists of careful surgical excision; consider tail amputation if multiple cysts endanger distal tail viability.

Digital and tail necrosis

Iguanas are prone to avascular necrosis of the toes and tail tip. This can be a sign of severe septicemia, mycotoxicosis, mycobacteriosis, mycosis, or mite infestation but most commonly results from retained molted skin causing avascular necrosis.[12] The latter is prevalent because of low humidity in captivity and is most frequent in smaller specimens. Differential diagnoses for swollen toes includes digital or joint infection, fracture, luxation (the most common etiology), and articular or periarticular gout or pseudogout.[146] Dental radiographs are useful to ascertain etiology. Iguanas whip their tails defensively, which can, in addition to retained molted skin, cause necrosis distally. For severely infected toes and tail tips, amputation with local anesthesia is indicated. Toes should be amputated flush with the foot and sutured. Tail tips should not be sutured because this inhibits regeneration.[12] The tail generally regenerates but is darker with finer scalation. In older iguanas, or with tails lost proximally, the tail may not regenerate. Nonsurgical manual amputation of the tail utilizing the natural fracture plane through the center of a vertebra causes little bleeding and is preferred to sharp amputation.[144] To do this, circumferentially inject lidocaine around the tail, anterior to the amputation site. The tail is then firmly grasped with both hands and bent sharply several times in a lateral plane with some rotational force until it snaps and separates. In large iguanas the skin may need to be incised but the vertebral body and muscles can still be manually separated. Light pressure for 5 minutes controls hemorrhage; the stump is bandaged for 3 days and then left open.

Egg retention and preovulatory follicles

Adult female iguanas often fail to lay any or all of their clutch in captivity. Eggs are produced regardless of male presence. Although there are many potential causes, the most common is lack of a suitable nesting site (see oviposition section in this chapter). In the wild, iguanas excavate large burrows, sometimes in communal nesting sites, and some travel considerable distances to return to them annually. Females are big enough for egg production when they are over 500 g, usually between 2 and 4 years of age, although large yearlings can also produce eggs. Peak incidence occurs in late fall through spring, which corresponds to the reproductive season in Panama. Females present hyporexic to anorexic with distended abdomens (figure 43). Normally, female iguanas are anorexic for 3 to 6 weeks prior to egg laying, probably because the large egg mass physically interferes with the gastrointestinal tract. The length of anorexia can guide management.

If hypocalcemic, the female may present collapsed with muscle tremors. Females may pace more, scratch or dig, try to get out of their cage, or be depressed. Gravid females should be handled carefully to avoid egg or oviductal rupture. A work-up of the female, with a complete blood count, plasma chemistry panel, and whole body radiographs, is recommended.

Females either have preovulatory follicles (much more common) or shelled eggs in the oviduct. The difference is important because follicles may be resorbed, whereas it is unlikely that shelled eggs can be resorbed and the female is likely to die from anorexia or egg-related coelomitis if the eggs are retained. In contrast to birds and chelonians, iguanas have soft-shelled eggs. Therefore radiographs delineate egg or follicle peripheries but rarely are distinct eggshells visible. Follicles tend to heavily overlap and flatten out in contact with one another and are more rounded than eggs. In contrast, oviductal eggs tend to be more dispersed with some distinct round or oval shapes visible (figure 44) and occasionally discernible eggshells.[165] It can be difficult to distinguish one from the other radiographically.

If the female is eating well or seems alert and vigorous and no major abnormalities are noted with physical examination and diagnostics (the female should be normocalcemic to hypercalcemic), the owner is encouraged to set up a nesting area (see oviposition section in this chapter). It is important that the female be disturbed as little as possible and be able to bask and behaviorally thermoregulate (see section on temperature in this chapter). Remember that normal iguanas go off food for 3 to 6 weeks prior to egg laying or 65 days after breeding. As long as the female is doing well, she can be given more time. Repeated diagnostics and good client communication are important. One should avoid letting the female's condition deteriorate enough that she becomes an anesthetic risk. Oxytocin has been unrewarding in the author's experience, but calcium injections (100 mg/kg 10% calcium gluconate IM q 6 hr) followed by oxytocin (1 to 10 IU/kg IM an hour after calcium injections) can be tried. Oxytocin is obviously of no benefit for preovulatory follicles. Surgery is recommended initially if the female has been anorexic for more than 6 weeks, if her condition has deteriorated, if serious abnormalities in blood or chemistry profiles or radiographs are present, or if the owner desires quick resolution of the situation. Correct hypocalcemia prior to surgery. Keep in mind that there is no clear set of rules for deciding between husbandry and medical management versus surgery; each case must be evaluated individually.

Ovariosalpingectomy is the simplest approach. A ventral paramedian incision, centered one-third of the distance from the rear legs to the front legs, avoids the large ventral abdominal vein. A midline incision is also feasible provided one takes care to avoid the ventral abdominal vein.[165] Iguanas lack an obvious coelomic (peritoneal) membrane, but it is initially easy to mistake the thin bladder wall for a coelomic membrane.

If the eggs are in the oviduct, the oviduct is exteriorized, mesovarium vessels are ligated, and then the posterior oviduct is ligated with two encircling absorbable sutures. The anterior oviduct is followed anteriorly to the infundibulum and either ligated or bluntly removed. The ovary is then carefully isolated and several large vessels running to it from the renal veins are ligated with 4-O synthetic absorbable suture or surgically stapled (much easier). Be careful to avoid the adrenal gland and the nearby large vessels. The same procedure is repeated on the other side. Totally removing the gravid oviduct and ovaries is much faster, easier, and induces less hemorrhage than individually removing eggs from the oviduct.

If preovulatory follicles are present, remove them as one would the ovaries, and leave the oviducts. Never leave the ovaries in place if the oviducts are removed, as the female may ovulate the following year. The author has consulted on several such cases that resulted in fatal egg yolk coelomitis (figure 45). The muscle layer is closed with 2-O absorbable suture and the skin closed with nonabsorbable suture or staples in a horizontal mattress pattern. Sutures are left in for at least 6 weeks, the belly can be wrapped for the first week. See Mader[165] for a more in-depth discussion of managing the gravid iguana.

Endoparasites and ectoparasites

Fecal examination is recommended. Ascarids (pinworms) are common and generally treated with fenbendazole granules or liquid by mouth (PO) biweekly for four treatments. Repeated fecal examinations are needed to determine efficacy. Some feel that pinworms are not harmful and may play a mechanical or enzymatic role in normal gut function.[166]

Red mites are the most common ectoparasites; ticks are rarely seen. Mites can cause considerable multifocal skin necrosis anywhere on the body and may be one cause of the "black skin disease" of iguanas described in the lay press (figure 46). Mites are difficult to detect in iguanas until present in massive numbers because they are very small and stay up under scale edges. They are best detected with magnification by looking up under scales for orangish areas or individual mites (figure 47). Skin scrapes or cytologic specimens gathered from an oil-soaked cotton-tipped applicators can also detect mites. Treatment is similar to that of snake mites (see section on diseases of snakes in chapter 5). Correct dehydration and stabilize the patient before insecticide usage. Rinsing in lukewarm water will remove large numbers of mites. Skin necrosis resolves once the mites are controlled; clinical discretion should determine the need for topical or systemic antibiotics and fluids. As with snake mites, lizard mites should not be tolerated in captivity.

Retained hemipenal plugs

Hemipenal waxy casts are commonly seen protruding from the cloaca in sexually mature males (figure 48). Waxy casts can be carefully pulled out while everting the hemipenes. Often the casts are palpable but not protruding from the cloaca.

Owner-directed seasonal male aggression

Mature male iguanas have been reported to attack female owners during their menstrual cycle, perhaps as a result of pheromones that the iguana can sense.[167] Male iguanas are also known to chase, bite, and even attempt to mate owners during the fall–winter breeding season in the absence of menstruating owners. Although we interpret this as an aberrant behavior, this is more likely normal behavior in an aberrant setting. Recall (from the introduction to this chapter) that adult male iguanas are known to be highly territorially aggressive during the breeding season.[131] Males start head bobbing more frequently and often eat much less at this time, both in captivity and in the wild. In the wild, large males patrol their territory, presumably in search of intruding males and receptive females.[131] Typically, territorial males approached most iguanas cautiously until the other iguanas fled, rebuffed the advances, or remained passive to allow breeding. Rodda[131] noted that occasionally territorial males seemed to recognize certain males at a distance. In these instances the male would fly at near-maximal speed toward the intruder, who would then run or jump out of the tree. This is strikingly similar to reports of captive iguanas streaking across the room to attack their owners.[168]

If we anthropomorphize, the iguana is simply viewing humans as potential rivals or mates. The iguana interprets certain individuals as males, which must be driven out of his territory. Others, especially those he approaches slowly, are interpreted as possible females, and he is waiting to see if they are receptive (a receptive female iguana is passive). With this in mind, several approaches to seasonal aggression are feasible. One is to cage the iguana and leave him alone as much as possible during the breeding season.[169] If the iguana is used to its cage, this is definitely advisable but still difficult (unless a shift cage has been built into the cage), because one still has to provide food and water (which is hazardous with a 5-foot lizard attacking you). Another alternative is to try to keep enough distance from the iguana so that you do not infringe on his territory. Several owners have told me this is usually about 10 to 15 feet away. Menstruating owners should probably avoid territorial males. Another approach is to stand your ground during attacks to show your iguana that you are the alpha male iguana.[168] Depending on the person, this may work or may be disastrous. The author hesitates to recommend this approach because iguana bites can be quite severe. Mature male iguanas are capable of amputating human fingers. Nonetheless, quickly picking up the iguana and returning it to its central territory seems to lessen its enthusiasm for attacking.[168] Another tactic is to take the iguana out of its familiar habitat and place it in a novel habitat. Barten[146] recommends changing the cage, changing the cage furnishings, moving the new cage to a new location, applying visual barriers, and removing any reflective surfaces. The new habitat may be unfamiliar enough that the iguana does not defend it.

Castration is often a veterinary recommendation, but it is currently unknown whether this decreases aggression. Some veterinarians feel that castration calms down an aggressive male iguana within several weeks and eventually abolishes aggressive behavior.[167] Others find no effect immediately after castration and anything from no effect to a somewhat less aggressive iguana a year later.[165] Keep in mind that the affects of castration may not be appreciated until the next breeding season. A familiar situation would be that of an aggressive male dog that may be slightly more manageable after castration but is still certainly an aggressive male dog.[146] Castration before puberty may lessen aggression in the future, based on a small number of cases.[146,165] Seasonal aggression may be worse at puberty and gradually decrease after several years of maturity. In any case, at this point, we do not really know how effective castration is. With these facts in mind, some iguana owners still elect to have castration done.

The surgical approach to castration is identical to that to ovarioectomy (see previously). Keep in mind that iguana testicles increase tremendously in size during the breeding season. If at all feasible, castrate them outside the breeding season to reduce surgical difficulty and risk.

Vascular clips are highly recommended because of the short distance (roughly 1 mm) between the right gonad and the vena cava.[165] Prepubertal castration will limit development of secondary sex characteristics that make male iguanas such impressive lizards.[165] Castration of mature males results in a color change from bronzish orange to the prepubertal bright lime green within a few weeks of castration.[167]

Other diseases

This has been a brief review of common iguana diseases in captivity. One should not infer from this that other diseases are not possible. Avoid tunnel vision. The astute clinician should pursue every opportunity to broaden their perspective and consider less common diseases.

For Further Reading

There are many good books on iguanas. Several the author consults are by Burghardt and Rand,[332] de Vosjoli,[137] Frye,[169] and Hatfield.[168]

4

Leopard Geckos

The leopard gecko, *Eublepharis macularius*, is a small fascinating lizard that in many ways represents the ideal starter lizard for the novice reptile keeper. Their catlike characteristics, soft velvety skin with leopard spots, docile temperament, hardiness, variable color patterns, and prolific nature make them very popular. They are native to western Asia, from eastern Iran into Afghanistan, southern Turkistan, Pakistan, and western India. Fortunately, they breed readily, so most are now captive born.

Leopard geckos do well in 10- to 20-gallon aquariums, with smooth aquarium stones (not sand or gravel) in the bottom, rocks for cover, and a water bowl. A combination nest box and hide box can be made from a shallow plastic container (any plastic container will do) with a hole cut in the lid or side and filled with 1 to 2 inches of moist (not wet or dry) vermiculite. Vermiculite is available from most plant stores, nurseries, and the plant sections of some grocery stores. The plastic container serves as a hide box that boosts humidity in a small area, to aid shedding in animals that otherwise need a dry environment, and provides an ideal egg-laying area for females. The geckos may eat the vermiculite but it passes through them harmlessly. As long as the vermiculite is kept moist, geckos should not have any problem with shed skin stuck on their toes. One male can be housed with several females, but not other males, as males will fight with one another.

Cage temperature should be 21 to 32°C (70 to 90°F). If the room temperature is not between these temperatures, heating pads, heat tape underneath the cage, or hot rocks inside the cage can boost temperatures. Use a thermometer to monitor temperature so that you do not have to guess what the temperature is. Leopard geckos can tolerate brief periods of cooler temperatures (4.5 to 18°C [40 to 65°F]) during the winter if they are in good health; this seems to be useful in breeding situations.

Geckos should be fed two to three times per week. Leopard geckos eat insects of all types such as grasshoppers, crickets, moths, flies, waxworms, and mealworms. As adults, many leopard geckos eat baby mice, which is recommended as an occasional substitute for their insectivorous fare. Overfeeding baby mice (more than two to three times per month) can lead to obesity. For more information, see the following section, feeding insectivorous reptiles and amphibians.

Leopard geckos are seasonally polyestrous. From late February to September females lay clutches of two eggs (rarely one) every 3 weeks for a total of 4 to 10 clutches. The longer day length seems to be the stimulus for breeding. Eggs can be incubated in a clean container with one part vermiculite to one part water by weight. Transfer the eggs to the incubator gently, keeping the same side up as when they were laid (see incubation section in chapter 1 for more information). At 27 to 29°C (80 to 85°F) the eggs should hatch in roughly 2 months. Temperature-dependent sex determination occurs in leopard geckos, with predominantly females produced between 28 and 29°C (82 and 84°F) and predominantly males above 30.5°C (87°F). Eggs fail to hatch well below 27°C (80°F) or above 32°C (90°F). Hatchlings begin feeding within 4 to 5 days on small crickets, waxworms, and mealworms. They have a banded pattern at first, which slowly transforms into the adult spotted pattern. If properly fed, they should reach adult size and breed within their first year. They can live 12 years or more.

Several problems are seen with leopard geckos. They seem more resistant to MBD than diurnal lizards but are not totally immune. The most common sign is a foreshortened and soft mandible and maxilla. Treatment is similar to that of green iguanas (see green iguana care in chapter 3). Without a moist hide box, digital dysecdysis frequently develops. Retained white skin is present on most digits and the tip of the tail. Without treatment the digits slough and can become infected. Soaking on damp paper towels is essential before carefully removing the stuck shed skin. Egg binding is also possible; the female may lay only one egg instead of two. Surgery is recommended; oxytocin does not seem helpful. Fine gravel, sand, or crushed walnut shells can cause intestinal impactions and rectal prolapse. Do not house leopard geckos on these substrates. Abdominal palpation will reveal the extent of the problem. Mineral oil enemas are useful, and the substrate should be changed. Skin lacerations heal very well if kept clean and treated topically every few days with triple antibiotic ointment. Most do not require sutures.

Feeding Insectivorous Reptiles and Amphibians

Insectivorous reptiles and amphibians are popular pet animals often purchased by well-meaning individuals who know little about their dietary needs. If fed one or two types of insects for several years, they may superficially appear normal until one day they die, for little apparent reason. If they are purchased before skeletal maturity, metabolic bone disease may rear its ugly head. How can we avoid both problems? To answer that question we must first appreciate the problem.

Insects have a negative ratio of calcium (Ca) to phosphorus (P); that is, they have much more P than they do Ca. For example, Ca-to-P contents of commonly fed insects, on an energy basis, are as follows: mealworms 0.1 to 1.2, crickets 0.2 to 2.6, waxworms 0.1 to 0.9, and grasshoppers 0.04 to 0.2 (the last listed as dry matter basis).[154,170] Reptiles that eat only insects do not get enough Ca in their diet, and over time this generally results in clinical to subclinical metabolic bone disease, especially in growing animals (figure 32).

Healthy Ca-to-P ratios in the diet of most vertebrates are generally considered to be one to two parts Ca for each part P. However, juvenile saltwater crocodiles selected natural diets with a Ca-to-P ratio of 6.7 to 1 (dry matter), whereas larger crocodiles ate diets with a Ca-to-P ratio of 1.85 to 1 (dry matter). The difference was explained by an ontogenic shift in prey selection. Smaller crocodiles ate more crabs and shrimp (which have calcium-rich shells) than larger crocodilians, which ate more rats, at the expense of crabs and shrimp.[170] Perhaps other reptiles undergoing rapid skeletal growth also select diets with a higher calcium content and shift to a lower calcium diet when skeletal growth slows. For example, both red-eared sliders[171] and green iguanas[133] are known to develop ontogenic shifts in diet. It was reported that pinhead crickets had a positive Ca-to-P ratio (1.6 to 1, dry matter basis) compared with adult crickets, having identical diets, with a Ca-to-P ratio of 1 to 4.[172]

The calcium content of insects can be improved by feeding them Ca-enriched diets and dusting them with Ca powder. Crickets fed rations with greater than 8% Ca developed positive Ca-to-P ratios after 2 days.[173] Rations of 5.7% Ca or higher were needed for 2 to 3 days to produce a positive Ca-to-P ratio in waxworms.[174] Zwart and Rulkens[175] and Frye and Calvert[176] discuss improving the nutritional content of mealworms and silk moth larvae, respectively. Frye[16,177] lists care and feeding for common feeder insects.

Fortified cricket diets are now commercially available (Ziegler Bros. Inc., 800-724-7370 or Fluker Farms, 800-735-8537). A mixture of 20% calcium carbonate and 80% nutritionally sound chick mash (by weight) is another example of a fortified insect diet.[178] These are not maintenance diets, but crickets are fine with them for several days, before being eaten, as long as they are moistened. Powdered monkey biscuits; dog, cat, or hermit crab food; and fresh fruits or vegetables do not have enough Ca in them to be useful for gut loading insects. Crickets that eat little in the pet store, or the reptile's cage, before being consumed are nutritionally bankrupt and detrimental over time.

Be aware that crickets will selectively eat mineral-poor fresh foods, such as fruits and vegetables, in preference to Ca-fortified rations if given the option.[173]

Another method of improving the Ca content of insects is to dust them with calcium. Suitable forms of Ca are calcium carbonate (oystershell, cuttlebone, or Tums® [SmithKline Beecham, Pittsburgh, PA]), lactate, citrate (all of which can be purchased in tablets from grocery stores, pharmacies, or health food stores), and gluconate. Calcium tablets can be crushed into powder with the back of a spoon or a mortar and pestle. The calcium should not have any P in it, as insects are already high in P and any additional P will make it difficult to achieve a positive Ca-to-P ratio. A wide variety of insect dusting powders are now available commercially; unfortunately, many of them still contain P and/or vitamin D—search for those that do not.

To dust insects, place them in a plastic bag with the Ca powder and shake. Dusted insects should be offered in amounts that can be quickly consumed because crickets groom themselves clean within half an hour to several hours.[173,178] Many geckos, particularly reproductively active females and young growing animals, will take powdered Ca directly from dishes left in the cage.

In addition to Ca, one must offer insectivores a wide variety of insects. Some commercially available insects are listed here.[154,178] Waxworms are larvae of the wax moth *Galeria mellonella* and are rich in fats and low in protein compared with other insects. Mealworms are larvae of the grain beetle *Tenebrio molitor* and have a highly chitinous exoskeleton, which has the potential for causing intestinal impaction in reptiles that feed exclusively on them. With a varied diet, this is not so much a concern, as most insectivores are chitinase producers. Mighty mealworms are larger larvae of the same grain beetle but have a higher fat and lower protein content. Super mealworms, *Xophobas morio*, are also available and are similar nutritionally to the mighty mealworm. Some advocate crushing the heads of larger mealworms before feeding so that they are less likely to perforate the stomach. Mealworms are the easiest of all insects to raise at home and also should be fed fortified chick mashes. Commercial crickets, *Acheta domesticus*, have a higher protein and lower fat content than most commercial insects. Fruit flies, *Drosophila melanogaster*, are useful for small frogs and neonatal chameleons and have the lowest fat content. Vestigial or wingless varieties are commonly used. Seasonally available insects such as moths, cicadas, flies, grasshoppers, bees (remove stingers), cockroaches, some caterpillars, and other insects should also be offered. At night insects can be collected around lights or concentrated with funnel traps. During the day sweep nets can collect insects from vacant lots or fields. When feeding wild-caught insects, make sure they have not been exposed to insecticides; if the insect is acting normally, chances are that it has not been. Sowbugs (pill bugs or roly polys) are terrestrial crustaceans (isopods) avidly taken by some chameleons and are a good source of Ca. In addition, many insectivores will eat baby mice (pinkies), hatchling finches, earthworms, slugs, and snails, which are excellent supplements (the latter items may pass trematodes). Snail shells are rich in calcium. For owners who object to live mice, pinkies can be purchased frozen from many pet stores and thawed in warm water just prior to feeding.

Insects should also be periodically dusted with multivitamins. For most vertebrates, vitamins A, D, and E should be in a ratio of 100:10:1.[154,178] Many bird and reptile multivitamins are poorly balanced with respect to these vitamins, as well as trace minerals. Human or domestic animal products (such as Centrum®, Lederle, American Cyanamid Co., Pearl River, NY) may actually be better balanced.[179] Note that multivitamins, enriched with minerals, do not contain enough calcium to prevent metabolic bone disease (irrespective of what the label implies).

Vitamins A and D, being fat soluble, are potentially toxic in excess. Oversupplementation with multivitamins often causes anorexia in chameleons that improves when multivitamins are curtailed. Limit multivitamin supplementation to once or twice a month by substituting multivitamins for the Ca powder when dusting. It is safer to allow the reptile to synthesize its own vitamin D, as needed, with exposure to ultraviolet light (discussed under ultraviolet light in chapter 1). Dierenfeld and Barker[178] believe that UV light may actually destroy excess vitamin A and prevent toxicity.[178]

See Allen and Oftedal,[180] Dierenfeld and Barker,[178] Donoghue,[179] and Donoghue and Langenburg[154] for current information on feeding insectivores.

5

Snakes

Taxonomy

Generalizations are difficult for such a diverse group. There is no substitute for good appreciation of natural history, but this is often beyond the curiosity of many veterinarians and more the responsibility of the owner. Nonetheless, take these generalizations as just that and realize that exceptions may occur. Excellent sources on captive care are listed in the references. Veterinarians should be aware of several of the more common groups of snakes.

Pythons and boas (boids) are large, primitive snakes that are always popular as pets. Boas give birth to live young, whereas pythons are egg layers. Boas have undivided subcaudal scales, in contrast to the paired subcaudals in pythons.

Colubrids are members of a large family, Colubridae, that inhabit every continent except Antarctica. Commonly kept colubrids include the milk snakes, king snakes, rat snakes, corn snakes, water snakes, garter snakes, ribbon snakes, racers, whip snakes, bull snakes, gopher snakes, pine snakes, green snakes, and many others. They are more advanced evolutionarily than boids in that they lack pelvic vestiges, the coronoid bone in the lower jaw, and a left lung. Be aware that certain rear-fanged colubrids such as boomslangs, twig snakes, red keel backs, and mangrove snakes are venomous.

The two major groups of venemous snakes include the fixed front-fanged (proteroglyphus) elapids and the folding front-fanged (solenoglyphus) viperids. Elapids include cobras, coral snakes, kraits, mambas, taipans, and a variety of Australian venemous snakes. Elapids, with their relatives the sea snakes, are some of the world's most venemous snakes. Viperids are divided into the Old World true vipers (vipers and adders) and the New and Old World pit vipers (rattlesnakes, cottonmouths, copperheads, bushmasters, vipers). Veterinarians should not consider working with venemous reptiles until they have had sufficient experience handling them.

Snake Care

Temperature

A thermal gradient within the cage is important to allow behavioral thermoregulation. Ambient temperature should range from a low of 21 to 24°C (70 to 75°F) at night to a high of 30 to 35°C (86 to 95°F) during the day, the lower temperatures for temperate colubrids and higher temperatures for tropical boids. The best way to achieve this is to warm the air temperature with a portable space heater. Provide a focal hot spot with a heating pad or heat tape, hot rock, or 15- to 75-watt incandescent light outside the tank (see temperature section in chapter 1). Hot rocks are not without problems and are generally discouraged, but they are better than no heat source at all. Heat sources inside the cage are a potential source of burns and should be used with caution. Direct contact with incandescent light bulbs is a sure recipe for thermal burns. Mounting lights in the center of the ceiling, well away from the sides, makes it difficult for a snake to bask directly on them. Vertical heat gradients within the room should also be used to advantage with cooler adapted species near the floor. A good-quality thermometer is important for monitoring temperatures; minimum–maximum thermometers are ideal. If signs of heat stress develop (pressing up against glass, retreating to the water bowl, avoiding hot spots), decrease the temperature immediately.

Humidity

Relative humidity should be 30% to 70% and can be increased by misting the cage with a spray bottle several times per week, using a humidifier, or providing a humid hide box. Plastic partially placed over the top will boost humidity, but it is important that the cage is ventilated as well. Low humidity can cause shedding problems, especially in tropical species. Xeric species often prefer lower humidity.

Housing

Snakes are best housed individually except for breeding groups. Different species should not be housed together; king snakes and some cobras are ophiophagic. Glass, plastic, or fiberglass aquariums do well for cages. Secure-fitting or weighted screen or pegboard tops are important because snakes (especially colubrids) can squeeze through very narrow openings. Wooden cages should be caulked and treated with an undercoat of water sealant and several overcoats of polyurethane, lacquer, enamel, or other waterproof paint. Make sure the cage is well aired (at least a week) before use. Melamine has become popular for cage and rack construction. To house large numbers of animals, breeders often use racks of shoe and sweater boxes. Hatchlings often do better in small shoe boxes than in larger aquariums. As a rough estimate, the cage should be almost as long as the snake and half as wide.[181]

A hide box, preferably plastic, should be present for all species. Nest boxes are important for breeding females. They can be made from plastic shoe or sweater boxes (or larger containers for big snakes), with a hole cut in the lid or side, and filled with damp sphagnum moss and vermiculite. Hardwood driftwood branches, polyvinyl chloride perches, or rocks are often useful. Snakes are not thought to require ultraviolet lighting, perhaps as a reflection of their fossorial past.

Substrates

Newspaper or butcher paper is an excellent choice for the bottom of the cage because it is cheap, easy to clean, and easily noticed when soiled or wet. Artificial turf or indoor–outdoor carpeting is less preferable because it has no absorptive qualities and can hide wetness. Having a second set of carpet allows one to be cleaned and dried while the other is in use. Aspen or pine shavings (not cedar shavings) and orchid bark work well. All need to be spot cleaned frequently and replaced periodically. Hatchlings can ingest small chips, which can be a hazard. Burrowing xeric species, such as sand boas, prefer sand or gravel. Burrowing humid species, such as rubber boas, prefer peat or sphagnum moss, cypress or pine mulch, or soil. Sand boas burrow to escape heat; thus heat provided from the bottom of the cage is inappropriate. Crushed corncob, walnut shells, and cat liter are not recommended because they are too dry and dusty.

Water

A water bowl should be present for all species, including large snakes. Keep the water clean; an easily removable water bowl is sensible. Built-in circulating water systems, such as a waterfall, may be aesthetically pleasing but are unsanitary. Those with large collections often opt for disposable plastic water bowls.

Feeding

Most snakes do well on a diet of rodents (exceptions will be mentioned). Rodents are nutritionally balanced and need no multivitamin supplementation if they are fed good-quality rodent chow prior to being fed. Although many owners of large pythons believe these snakes need additional vitamins, there is little evidence to support this (faster growth is not always correlated with long-term health). Avoid diseased, starving, or wild-caught rodents because they can transmit diseases and internal or external parasites to the snake. Rodents should be humanely killed or stunned before offering them to the snake so that they do not injure the snake. Rodents can inflict serious bites to the eyes, mouth, head, or body that may abscess or even kill the snake. Left unattended and hungry, it is common for rodents to chew on the tail and dorsum of snakes and cause extensive damage without any self-defense from the snake (figure 49). Occasionally, finicky or recently acquired snakes may need a live rodent to induce feeding. If water and food are provided, the rodent can be left in the cage for less than 12 hours, but one should be alert for problems. Most snakes can eventually be converted to killed or stunned rodents. Given the choice, snakes actually prefer thawed rodents over freshly killed ones.[182] Mice and rats are the staple for smaller snakes; large specimens eat rabbits and chickens. Gerbils, hamsters, guinea pigs, and pigeons also can be used. Chicken legs are not a nutritionally balanced staple diet but are a good source of *Salmonella.*

Garter snakes and ribbon snakes (*Thamnophis*) eat fish, frogs, earthworms, and sometimes baby mice (especially if rubbed with fish). Water snakes (*Nerodia*) are semiaquatic snakes that eat goldfish, minnows, shiners, trout, and smelt. Except for trout, the mentioned fish contain thiaminases, which can induce thiamine deficiencies in snakes fed them exclusively. Supplementation with brewer's yeast, warming fish up to 80°C (176°F), or feeding a balanced diet should prevent thiamine deficiencies.[183] Fish can be floated in the water bowl to stimulate feeding.

Handling

Large snakes can inflict serious painful bites with razor-sharp teeth and should be handled with respect. Reticulated pythons, blood pythons (*P. curtus*) and rock pythons (*P. sebae*), Caribbean boas (*Epicrates* spp.), tree boas, and anacondas (*Eunectes* spp.) are notoriously snappy. Most wild-caught snakes bite initially but quickly calm down with handling. Veterinary examination may induce normally docile snakes to bite. Most boids form their neck into an S-shaped coil prior to striking. Never approach a snake's head from in front if it is coiled to strike. Draping a towel over the head, restraining the head from outside the bag, or slowly working a hand up the body to the head avoids bites. Most bites are defensive and the snake releases immediately. If the snake bites and holds on, squirting a little alcohol into the mouth will often make the snake let go. If this fails, one can carefully pry off the snake's jaws. Remember that snakes have posteriorly recurved teeth that must be pulled cranially to release. Simply pulling the jaws out breaks teeth, tears flesh, and results in much more damage to all parties.

It is incumbent upon veterinarians to observe and advise owners of large snakes to heed the guidelines offered by the American Federation of Herpetoculturists[184,185] for giant snakes (summarized as follows):

1. Snakes should not be displayed in public where people would not reasonably expect to see them. Do not force snakes on those who might not want to see them (which are often other pets and owners in the waiting room).

2. Transport snakes in a safe manner that precludes escape and keeps them out of sight. For example, put the snake in a bag and put the bag in a box or in another bag.

3. Snakes over 8 feet in length should be kept in a secure cage with some sort of locking mechanism. The cage should be inside a room with a door, so that in the unlikely event that the snake got out of the cage, it would still be contained within the room.

4. When handling any large constrictor over 8 feet or 30 pounds, a second person should be present or within calling distance. This is extremely important and should be observed by even the most experienced snake handler.

5. Minors should seek parental consent before obtaining giant snakes to ensure proper housing, maintenance, and supervision. No store should sell giant snakes without providing local regulations and guidelines for responsible maintenance.

6. Establish a set feeding routine that is distinct from your cleaning or handling routines. The author recommends using a shift cage for feeding, such as a plastic trash can with locking handles and numerous ventilation holes. When feeding, assist the snake into the shift cage with a large snake hook. Inside the shift cage can be the prekilled prey item. Avoid offering prey with one's own hand. Do

not enter a snake's cage with a prey item on you or already in the cage. Avoid cleaning or handling snakes after handling prey or during feeding.

7. Keep in mind that, just as with dogs, owners of large constrictors may be held liable for the treatment and trauma inflicted on someone by their snake's bite.

Hibernation

Hibernation is not without risk but is recommended for most temperate species that normally hibernate. This includes most captive colubrids and excludes tropical boids. Hold snakes without food for 2 weeks before cooling to allow all food to be digested. Then discontinue heating sources and keep the snake at room temperature (15 to 21°C [60 to 70°F]) for another week. The snake is then ready to enter hibernation. Its cage should be transferred to a draft-free dry area, with little light, that can be kept between 7 and 15°C (45 and 60°F), such as a basement, garage, back porch, or north- or east-facing closet, window, wall, or wine cellar. Freezing should be avoided. Consistent temperatures above 15°C (60°F) are too warm, and instead of hibernating, the snake will metabolize its body fat and slowly starve. A minimum–maximum thermometer is useful for monitoring temperatures throughout hibernation; cold snaps may make the hibernaculum too cold. The snake can be hibernated in its cage or a plastic sweater box. The cage should not rest directly on cold flooring; newspaper under the cage provides enough insulation. Clean water should always be available. If the snake starts to shed during hibernation, warm it up, allow it to shed, and then return it to the hibernaculum. Snakes should be checked every 1 to 2 weeks. If signs of respiratory illness (excess mucus in mouth, gurgling, nasal discharge) develop, warm the snake up to 26.5 to 32°C (80 to 90°F) and begin antibiotic treatment immediately. Length of hibernation depends on local temperatures, the animal's condition, and the owner's preference. Three to five months is average.

Hibernation is important for stimulating breeding in colubrids. In the spring, upon emergence from hibernation, the snake should be warmed up (24 to 30°C [75 to 85°F]) for a few days and fed a small meal. Prey items can be increased gradually in size over the next several feedings. Females have ravenous appetites and should be fed as much as they will eat to prepare them for breeding. Some males may be so focused on breeding that their appetite lags behind that of females or they refuse to feed. Generally, males start feeding later in the breeding season.

Shedding (ecdysis)

Shedding is more frequent during periods of increased growth, temperature, and food consumption or if skin disease or injury is present. Younger animals shed more frequently, usually about once a month. The skin takes on an opaque or dull color, first on the ventral tail and then spreading anteriorly. Once at the head level, the snake's eyes become milky blue and are said to be opaque. While they are opaque, new epithelium is being rapidly produced underneath the older epithelium. It is important not to handle the snake at this time, because the newly forming epithelium is fragile. If the old epithelium is rubbed off before the new epithelium has matured, permanent scarring can result. It is the author's practice not to examine snakes while opaque; rather, advise the owner to bring the snake back after shedding is complete. Exceptions to this rule include any life-threatening illness; see the section on lower respiratory tract infections later in this chapter for related information. After the eyes have been opaque for a few days, they clear, indicating that the new epithelium is mature. The snake should begin shedding anywhere from 2 to 10 days after the eyes have cleared. It is vital to provide water and keep the cage more humid during shedding (see the following section).

Dysecdysis

Snakes with stuck shed skin can look quite serious (figure 50), but are fine once the stuck shed is off (figure 51). Difficulty shedding is often a result of low humidity, particularly in boids, and can be easily managed through changes in husbandry. After the eyes clear and until the snake has completely shed, it is important to keep the cage humid by spraying it daily with lukewarm (24°C [75°F]) water. A water bowl, big enough to allow soaking, should be present, as well as some rocks, branches, or cage furniture to rub against as an aid in removing the old skin.

It is abnormal if the old skin has not all come off within 24 hours of the onset of shedding. Usually, heavily spraying the snake and cage will allow it to shed in 1 or 2 days. If this does not work, soak the snake in a container just big enough to contain the snake with a brick and just enough water to reach two-thirds of the way up the side of the snake. Be sure the container is not too large and the water not too deep, or the snake may start swimming and drown. A safer alternative is to put the snake in a pillowcase with a wet towel. In either case, after 30 to 60 minutes (or longer if possible) remove the snake and gently peel off the stuck shed starting rostrally and working caudally. Once onto the body, one can slowly peel the skin posteriorly with an encircling thumb and forefinger while allowing the snake to pull slowly forward and out of its shed skin. Resist the temptation to remove portions of stuck shed out of sequence, as this will make it harder to remove the entire skin later. Make sure you remove all skin, especially from the head and tail. Check the shed skin to see if the eye caps were removed. With either method, make sure the air temperature stays warm (24 to 30°C [75 to 85°F]) so that the snake does not become chilled in the damp environment.

Retained spectacles or eye caps should be obvious (figure 52). Little bits of retained shed skin are visible periocularly and it is difficult to get a clear view of the eye because of the shed stuck on it. Simple wrinkling of the eye cap is not a retained spectacle! If there is any doubt, it is probably not a retained spectacle. Check the shed skin for eye caps. If you are still unsure, the safest alternative is to wait until the next shed, at which time the spectacles should come off. If a retained eye cap is not present and one starts manipulating the outer surface of the spectacle, serious corneal damage is possible (figure 53). Owners often seek veterinary assistance at this point; be careful not to do further harm.

If retained spectacles are present, soak the snake for several hours or apply ophthalmic lubricant until the spectacle softens. Retained spectacles should come off easily on rubbing a Q-tip over them or gently teasing off some of the retained periocular shed with a pair of fine forceps or fingernails.

For Further Reading

For further information on the natural history or husbandry of snakes, see Applegate,[186] Barker and Barker,[187] de Vosjoli,[184,185,188] de Vosjoli et al.,[189] Greene,[190] Kaulfield,[191] McEchern,[192] Mehrtens,[193] Perlowin,[194] Ross and Marzec,[195] Rossi,[183] Rossi and Rossi,[181] and Shine.[196]

Basic Medical Techniques for Snakes

Physical examination

As discussed in the section on shedding, snakes generally should not be examined while shedding or a few days after eating (or they may regurgitate). Physical examination begins at the head and moves caudally. Check the nares, labial pits, and periorbitally for any mites, ticks, or retained shed skin. Mites are frequently found between scales in the gular area or around the vent (figure 53). The oral cavity should always be examined. Two disposable cotton-tipped applicators (5-inch-long Q-tips) are gently forced through the front of the mouth and spread apart in the rear of the mouth. Gentle pressure exerted anteriorly against the inner rostral maxillary teeth elicits a gap response that allows gentle but thorough examination of the oral cavity, even in large snakes (figure 55). Many clinicians prefer soft rubber spatulas or other specula, which is fine as long as they are used carefully and disinfected with each usage. The oral mucosa should be pale pink (many species have darker pigments present) with little mucus. Petechiae, yellow or green areas of necrosis, are early signs of infectious stomatitis (figure 56). There should be no mucus or discharge from the glottis or nares in normal snakes, but these exudates are often present with respiratory tract infections. In respiration there can be a slight normal wheeze, especially with exhalation, which is much more apparent the larger the snake gets. Gurgling is abnormal. Respiratory sounds are often normally increased prior to shedding. Retained shed skin in the nares can cause high-pitched respiratory noises (almost a whistle) or occlusion.

From the head, slowly run a thumb down the ventrum while deeply palpating. In smaller snakes, one sequentially feels the trachea and the heart in the cranial third of the snake; the liver and stomach (if ingesta is present) in the middle third; and gallbladder, ova, kidneys, and sometimes uric acid accumulations in the cloaca in the caudal third. The gallbladder may be in the caudal middle third, depending on the species. Palpation is difficult without anesthesia in larger snakes. Other structures are generally not palpable. Cryptosporidiosis often results in a palpable gastric wall thickening. Epaxial grooves should not be obvious in the caudal half of snakes of good body weight (figure 57). In underweight snakes, the epaxial grooves extend farther caudally and the ribs are prominent. With extreme cachexia, the vertebral bodies become obvious and the skin tears easily.

Examine the cloaca for mites, ticks, anal sac or hemipenal infections, or signs of inflammation. Feces can often be gently squeezed from the caudal third of small snakes after first expressing urinary wastes. This should be done very carefully without undue pressure. Feces can be examined after centrifugation and concentration in solutions denser than water (such as zinc sulfate). Nematode and cestode ova are easily detected in this manner. Protozoans are better detected with cloacal or colonic washes or wet mounts of fresh feces. Colonic washes are obtained by carefully pressing a ball-tipped tube anteriorly and ventrally through the colonic sphincter into the colon, injecting a little saline, and then aspirating. Small mucoid debris collected can immediately be observed for protozoans. Always weigh and sex the patient. See Barten[197] for more information on physical examination.

Sexing

Hatchling and juvenile snakes can be sexed, with practice, by gently arching the spine dorsal and caudal to the cloaca, while rolling one's thumb posterior to anterior and popping out one hemipenis (sometimes two; figure 58). Inserting an appropriate-sized probe caudal to the cloaca and then counting the depth of subcaudal scale penetration is another easy method of sex determination. Females probe less than three or four subcaudals, whereas males, because of their hemipenes, probe five to six or more subcaudals. Be careful; undue force may pierce the caudal cloacal wall and make a female appear to be a male! It is normal for female colubrids to bleed slightly after probing. Males also tend to have longer tails and consequently higher subcaudal scale counts and larger remnants of the pelvic girdle known as spurs.

Venipuncture

In colubrids and viperids, the ventral coccygeal vein is accessible as in lizards. In boids, tail bleeding is difficult; therefore cardiocentesis is much more widely practiced. Cardiac puncture involves a low level of mortality if multiple attempts do not overly traumatize the heart,[120] but it is prudent to warn clients that, in rare instances, death can result. The heart can be localized by palpation or watching for it beating ventrally, within 20% to 40% of the distance between the snout and vent.[198] Stabilize the heart by pushing anteriorly with a thumb at the apex, and have a second person place a forefinger anterior to the heart base (figure 59). The second person should also restrain the snake; anesthesia is recommended, especially for large animals. The heart is then punctured with a 22- to 25-gauge heparinized needle, attached to a 1- to 6-cc syringe, through the apex of the single ventricle. Clear fluid initially indicates pericardial fluid contamination; remove the needle and try again.[199]

The dorsal and ventral buccal veins can be used to collect blood from a needle hub with microhematocrit tubes,[200,201] but it is difficult to collect large volumes as the veins collapse easily.

Diseases of Snakes

Anorexia

Anorexia is the most common presenting complaint of snakes and is a symptom of disease but not a disease in and of itself.[202] Before one can decide whether the snake is truly anorexic, one must know how often snakes eat. Sedentary snakes feed much less frequently than snakes with higher metabolic rates. Hatchlings and breeding females should feed several times per week; juveniles and adults usually feed once or twice a week. Gravid or pregnant females may cease eating. Larger boids that consume large prey items (such as rabbits) may feed only every 3 to 6 weeks. More often than not, anorexia is related to husbandry, but it is also a nonspecific symptom of most diseases. A good history should discern environmental temperature and cage setup, feeding practices, length of anorexia, whether intermittent or constant, and whether regurgitation or any other problems are present. Recent acquisitions, too cool environmental temperature (especially at night), frequent handling, too large prey or a change in prey, shedding, presence of other snakes in the cage, decreased photoperiod in the winter for temperate colubrids, and mites can all result in anorexia. Many snakes refuse food a week or so prior to shedding. Thus, the initial steps in working up an anorexic snake are a good history and physical examination, which give one a feel for presence or absence of disease. Almost any disease can cause anorexia. If the health status is uncertain, basic diagnostics might include a fecal examination, blood work, or radiographs. For snakes that appear healthy on physical examination, some simple husbandry tricks often entice feeding (see the following discussion).

Wild-caught ball pythons, *Python regius*, are frequently presented for not eating. In the wild they are specialized nocturnal predators that undergo periodic fasts when food is not available. Their natural prey species are not available in captivity, so it takes a bit of coercing to get them to try new prey. Ball pythons are relatively shy snakes. Handling, even infrequently, may cause a wild-caught ball python not to feed. The longer the snake has been handled, the longer it will be before it begins feeding. In the natural habitat ball pythons spend much time underground, in jumping mouse burrows; thus providing several hide boxes is a good management technique. Clay flower pots seem preferred. Ball pythons typically go off feed during the winter breeding season. Females do not feed while gravid or when brooding eggs.[187] Imported ball pythons are typically off feed between November and April.[182]

Adult ball pythons often do not begin feeding for 6 to 12 months after importation. As long as the snake is not seriously underweight, this should not cause problems. An exception is hatchling ball pythons. Hatchlings can starve to death within several months if not fed. However, hatchlings are generally captive born and thus have less problems with eating. During the initial acclimation period for adult ball pythons, correct husbandry and stop handling the snake. A thorough physical examination is important to evaluate health and discuss management options with the owner. Make sure the ambient cage temperature is above 24°C (75°F) at night and warmed to 30 to 32°C (85 to 90°F) during the day with a localized hot spot up to 35°C (95°F). Wild-caught ball pythons are heavily parasitized and should be wormed with fenbendazole and praziquantel[203,204] and treated for ectoparasites if present. Offer food when the snake seems active or just after shedding. An indication that the snake is ready to feed is that it starts sticking its head out of the entrance of the hide box. Fuzzy mice, adult mice, or fuzzy rats should be left in the cage overnight (see diet section in this chapter for precautions). Try to disturb the snake as little as possible when putting prey in the cage; warn the owner not to try to watch the snake eat or check on it until the next day. Movement outside the cage is enough disturbance to make these reclusive snakes not want to eat that night. If the snake has not eaten by morning, remove the prey and try again a few days later or offer different prey. If the snake does not eat live food, try a freshly killed mouse, rat, gerbil, or hamster in a variety of different sizes or colors. Another technique that occasionally works is to create a rodent nest by placing some rodent nest material and feces in the unoccupied hide box with a few baby rodents. At night, when the ball python is active, it may discover the nest and eat the prey. Others have had success placing the snake, with a fuzzy rat, in a brown paper bag overnight.[187] Above all, one must have patience; it may be months before the python begins feeding. If the preceding techniques fail or the snake appears thin, several force-feedings often induces voluntary feeding. Once the snake has fed four times on its on, limited handling can be undertaken as long as the snake continues eating.

Colubrid anorexia is another story entirely. Many temperate colubrids naturally cease feeding in the late summer (as early as August), fall, or winter and do not feed again until spring. Considerable variation is to be expected even with conspecific animals under identical conditions. Shorter day length seems to be more of a driving force than environmental temperature. If the snake has a good body weight and appears healthy, hibernation is recommended (discussed in section on snake care in this chapter). Snakes with signs of illness, recent illness, surgery, trauma, or severe emaciation should not hibernate. A fecal examination several months prior to hibernation is useful.

It can be difficult to get some hatchling colubrids to feed, but they have enough yolk stored to last them a few months. Resist the temptation to force-feed them until all efforts to get them to feed voluntarily have been exhausted. They should be transferred to plastic shoe boxes with newspaper, a water bowl, a hide box (a clay saucer with a hole chipped in one side works well), and adequate cage temperature. Minimize handling until they are feeding well.

Once set up correctly, several tricks work well to get hatchling snakes to feed (some also work for adults). The simplest approach is to place a pinkie (try both live and killed) in the hide box overnight, without disturbing the snake. Attempt this several times or offer food in the morning. If this fails, an extremely successful technique is called "braining." The technique is gruesome; however, the means certainly justify the end result. Many individuals will steadfastly refuse pinkies, then immediately devour the first "brained" pinkie offered. To do this, a pinkie is killed and a small amount of brain is squeezed onto the pinkie's snout through a skull incision or forced out through the nostrils. The brained pinkie is then presented to the snake or left near the snake in the cage overnight. Once the snake starts tongue flicking and picks up the brain scent, it seems to reflexively eat the pinkie.

If braining fails, other options exist. More aggressive species sometimes can be induced to strike and coil around a killed baby mouse. If one then carefully closes the cage and exits, so as not to disturb the snake, the snake will often eat if undisturbed for several hours. Sometimes this works after two or three attempts. A brained pinkie will sometimes be taken in this manner. For very small arboreal snakes, it often helps to cut the pinkie in half; snakes that drop a full pinkie will often hold onto and consume half.

Lizard-eating species, such as some milk snakes and king snakes, will take pinkies scented with lizards. To do this, kill a pinkie, wash off its scent with warm dishwashing liquid, and then dry it off. Take some skin or limbs from a dead lizard, or grind up some lizard until mushy, and rub this all over the washed pinkie (particularly the head). Leave this with the snake overnight. If that fails, but the snake will eat lizards, try tying a pinkie to the lizard and offer the lizard to the snake. On subsequent feedings, offer less and less lizard, until only a little lizard is needed to stimulate feeding. Use just enough cotton thread to attach the two and trim any loose ends. Some species can be enticed to feed with a rodent nest.

Some snakes can be induced to eat with a few doses of metronidazole at 100 mg/kg.[12] In particular, anorexic juvenile boa constrictors and other boids respond beautifully to this treatment.

If all these methods fail, have the owner try different prey items. A combination of methods sometimes works. Find out what the given species naturally feeds on. Force-feeding should be a last resort and can kill small snakes, so be careful doing it. A commercial force-feeding pump is available that macerates pinkies and allows them to be stomach tubed (Pinkie Pump, BJ Specialties, 2802 Melody Lane, Columbia, MO 65203, 314-442-8558).

Regurgitation

Regurgitation is common in boids and is a symptom of other disease, rather than a disease itself.[202] Common causes include handling the snake too soon after feeding (avoid handling for several days after feeding), parasites (particularly protozoans), suboptimal environmental temperature, or too large a meal. Less common causes include bacteria, viruses (especially paramyxovirus and inclusion body disease virus), foreign bodies, and organ system failure. Juvenile boa constrictors are especially prone to regurgitation. Wild-caught emerald tree boas, *Corallus canina*, are prone to a regurgitation syndrome of unknown cause that may be terminal. However, one should still attempt to rule out treatable causes of regurgitation. Typical symptoms include irregular coiling, with the stomach area loosely looped over a branch and the posterior coils wrapped tightly around the branch, dullness and inelasticity of skin, runny stools, and weight loss.[205]

Work-up of regurgitating snakes first includes a thorough review of husbandry and history, then careful physical examination. If environmental causes are not suspected, examine feces, stomach, cloacal or colonic washings, or the surface slime from regurgitated food items for evidence of parasites. Large numbers of protozoans are often found in regurgitating snakes and seemingly respond to metronidazole. If parasites are not obvious, consider acid-fast stains for *Cryptosporidium* or acid-fast bacteria. If *Cryptosporidium* oocytes or other parasites are not detected, consider symptomatic treatment with metronidazole. Plain and contrast radiographs, chemistry panels, complete blood counts, and bacterial culture and sensitivity may be indicated for further work-up.

Lower respiratory tract infections

Respiratory tract infections are much more common in boids than in colubrids. Often the history will reveal an episode of chilling; temperatures below 21°C (70°F), even for a short time, can result in pneumonia. Clinical signs may include any or all of the following: gurgling respiratory sounds, increased mucus in the oral cavity or glottis, open-mouthed breathing (especially with clogged nares), anorexia, and holding the head and neck elevated at a 45-degree or greater angle (figure 60). Useful diagnostics include tracheal-wash aerobic and anaerobic cultures with antibiotic sensitivities. Cytology of glottal discharges may reveal evidence of nematodes or their eggs. The most important aspect of treatment is raising the environmental temperature to 26.5 to 32°C (80 to 90°F). Pending sensitivity results, good injectable antibiotics include enrofloxacin, ceftazidime, and amikacin. If cultures indicate that anaerobes are present, add carbenicillin. Coupage with the snake's head held ventrally may also help to expel mucous secretions. Antibiotic therapy should continue for a minimum of 3 weeks, or at least a week after clinical signs resolve. The author also routinely treats snakes with pneumonia for nematodes with ivermectin every 2 weeks for four treatments. See Murray[206] for a good review of anatomy and treatment of respiratory tract disease.

Suspected respiratory tract infection is a frequent presenting complaint for many large snakes, yet the majority of these patients are not sick. Large boids normally have an audible smooth expiratory wheeze that becomes more noticeable as the snake gets larger. This is not to be confused with gurgling. Owners note this wheezing and mistake it for a respiratory tract infection. Shed skin stuck in the nares can also increase respiratory sounds. In addition, many snakes develop increased respiratory sounds, ventral erythema, and anorexia in the days prior to shedding. Generally, the author recommends a checkup after shedding. Although it is potentially detrimental to examine opaque snakes, in certain instances it may be prudent to check carefully for excessive mucus in the mouth and listen with the open bell of a cardiac stethoscope for gurgling tracheal noises. If the snake truly has a respiratory tract infection, it is fairly obvious; when in doubt, wait until the snake sheds. It is rare for a snake to be consistently feeding if it does have a respiratory tract infection.

Infectious stomatitis

Early signs of infectious stomatitis, mouth rot, or canker include oral petechiae and increased mucus in the mouth. The petechiae progress to areas of white, yellow, gray, or green oral mucosa with swelling and accumulated cellular debris (figure 56). Mild cases respond well to increased environmental temperature, gentle daily topical disinfection, and topical antibiotics. Treatment of advanced cases involves aggressive débridement of necrotic tissue (including bone) under general anesthesia, a culture for antibiotic selection, injectable and local antibiotics, and careful rinsing (see below). Radiographs are indicated if bone involvement is suspected; dental radiographs work well.

Mucus in the oral cavity can be rinsed out with warm water and the mouth flushed, painted, or sprayed with 1% chlorhexidine diacetate (Nolvasan, 2% scented disinfectant, Fort Dodge) or tamed iodine. Extreme care should be taken to prevent the snake from aspirating any mucus or rinse when the glottis opens during inhalation. Topical treatment with gentamicin sulfate (Gentocin ophthalmic solution or ointment, Schering-Plough) is also useful. Initially, the mouth should be cleaned once or twice daily, with treatment tapering as the infection resolves and healing begins. Treatment requires two or more persons. In large snakes gauze stirrups are useful in keeping the mouth open and less traumatic than solid specula. Débridement usually lasts a week in severe cases, but be careful not to traumatize the mouth inadvertently with overzealous treatment. Severe cases often require several months of intensive treatment, mild cases a week or two. Most snakes will not eat during treatment. If the snake has a good body weight, this is acceptable, but if the snake is thin force-feeding is indicated so that an adequate immune response can be generated. Maintain hydration as well. Severe infectious stomatitis should be treated for several days in the hospital with continued treatment after this by the owner and weekly rechecks. The prognosis is good for most cases, but permanent facial deformity of the anterior rostrum may lead to future exposure gingivitis. Warn owners that this is not recurrence of mouth rot.

Mites

Mites are a common problem in snakes and can transmit bacteria, blood parasites, and perhaps even viruses between reptiles, in addition to draining considerable amounts of serum. They cause intense discomfort to the host and can weaken the reptile enough that secondary infections, generalized ill health, and even death may result (such as with heavy flea infestations in mammals). Mites should be eliminated whenever present, even if only a single mite is observed. Snakes infected with mites spend more time soaking in the water bowl and have difficulty shedding. Mites are best seen periocularly, between gular scales (figure 54), around the cloaca, or drowned in the water bowl.

There are more recommendations for treatment of mites than for any other malady in reptiles. This reflects the fact that mites (or perhaps more accurately, their eggs) are difficult to eradicate and treatment failure is common. Insecticidal sprays are by far the most effective treatment, but there is a fine line between efffective treatment and toxicosis. Currently the author is using a dilute pyrethroid spray (5 [0.007%] to 15 ml [0.002%] Permectrin II, Boehringer Ingelheim

Animal Health, in 710 ml of tap water) every 2 weeks for three treatments to eliminate mites.[207]

Snake mites lay their eggs off the host, so the environment, as well as the snake, must be treated. This undoubtably explains widespread treatment failure, as many past recommendations focused on treating only the snake. Mites also spread rapidly throughout a collection or even a building. If in doubt about the extent of the problem, treat the entire collection. As a minimum, consider treating all in contact cages.

Treatment is certainly labor intensive. First the entire cage (inside and out) must be cleaned with warm soapy water, then rinsed to remove all waste material. Mites especially favor the cracks and seams in cages for egg laying. Remove all cage furniture, such as water bowls and plastic hide boxes, and clean them thoroughly. Discard any wooden hide boxes or branches, as mites often lay eggs deep within them. Discard any substrates, especially any soil or moist substrate. When the cage is clean and dry, spray it thoroughly with dilute Permectrin spray and allow the cage to air dry once more. Line the bottom of the cage with newspaper. Within the next 12 hours any mites that escaped cleaning should die from the Permectrin spray.

Once the cage is treated, the snake can be treated. Spray the entire snake with the dilute spray, starting around the head and working down the back and then up the belly. Include the labial pits, if present, and around the eyes. Avoid getting spray in the snake's mouth; a little does not cause problems. When the snake has been thoroughly sprayed, lightly run a paper towel down to its length to absorb excess spray, and return it to the cleaned, dried, treated cage. It is important that the cage be well aired out before returning the snake to the cage so that the fumes do not overwhelm the snake. Pyrethrin and pyrethroid vapors can be quite toxic. Withhold water for several days so that the snake cannot soak off the spray. Spray the snake and its cage again at 2 and 4 weeks (for a total of three treatments) with freshly made diluted spray. If the snake is getting ready to shed, wait until after it sheds for treatment. If the snake is very ill, thin, or dehydrated, consider supportive care prior to treatment. The key to sucessful treatment is thorough cleaning and following through with all three treatments. See Mader[208] and Stahl[209] for more information on mites and treatment.

Inclusion body disease of boids

Inclusion body disease (IBD) is a serious, fatal, suspected retroviral infection of boids. Herpetologists may refer to this as stargazing disease, boid encephalitis, or twisty.[210] The disease has been seen in large collections in Europe, Africa, and the United States for the last 25 years.[211,212] See Schumacher et al.[212] for detailed clinicopathologic findings. In boa constrictors the first signs include intermittent regurgitation and sometimes head tremors, which progress to dysecydysis, chronic regurgitation, and anorexia. Regurgitation may not be present in all cases. Boas lose weight and may have clogged nares, stomatitis, or pneumonia. The disease rapidly progresses to include central nervous symptoms such as disorientation, disequilibrium (corkscrewing of head and neck, holding the head unnaturally, rolling onto the back without a righting reflex), star gazing (a blank stare off to nowhere) and opisthotonus (figure 61).[212,213] In Burmese pythons, neurologic signs arose earlier and were more frequent and pronounced than in boa constictors (most likely because of a more severe and diffuse inflammatory cell infiltrate in the brain).[210,212] Regurgitation was rare in Burmese pythons; anorexia was not. Pythons often show a progressive loss of motor function, especially in the rear half, which may lead to bloating.[213] Boids may hold their tongues out longer than normal while tongue flicking. Boa constrictors acutely infected (< 2 months) demonstrated leukocytosis with lymphocytosis, compared with chronically infected (> 2 months) boas with lymphopenia.[212] Jacobson[214] reported less typical neurologic signs in the past few years and more stomatitis, pneumonia, and lymphoproliferative disorders in boa constrictors. Keep in mind that if the snake survives long enough, neurologic signs may wane but the snake will never feed voluntarily again.

Plasma biochemical values and gross necropsies were unremarkable except for some splenic and pancreatic atrophy, pneumonia, and white circular nodules on the surface of the kidneys in a few snakes.[212] Basophilic (Giemsa stain) or eosinophillic (hematoxylin-eosin stain), intracytoplasmic inclusions, 1 to 4 μm in size, were seen in most epithelial organs of some snakes (hence the name), whereas others had less inclusions restricted to the central nervous system.[212] Mites are suspected to be a vector, as most epidemics also involved mite problems.[212] Direct contact between snakes or contaminated bedding, mating, and vertical transmission are other possible means of transmission.[213] Research planning is under way at the University of Florida to develop a serologic test but this may take several years (or more, depending on funding). Suspected cases can sometimes be diagnosed by the presence of inclusion bodies in red or white cells[215] or from renal, hepatic, gastric, pancreatic, or esophageal tonsillar crypt biopsies with complete blood counts. Absence of inclusions does not rule out disease.[210]

Affected snakes either die acutely or starve slowly after several years of anorexia. The author has seen suspected cases kept alive for long periods with force-feeding. As infected snakes are chronic carriers and recovery has not been reported, euthanasia is recommended. However, euthanasia based solely on clinical signs may lead to misdiagnosis, as other central nervous system diseases can present with similar signs.[213] In the past, many chronic pneumonias nonresponsive to antibiotics may have been IBD.

Ophidian paramyxoviral infection

This is undoubtedly the most dangerous disease facing large collections of snakes. This virus was first discovered after a Swiss outbreak that resulted in death of more than 25% of over 400 fer-de-lance (*Bothrops atrox*) in 1973.[216] Since then, there have been numerous die-offs of viperids, especially crotalids, in many large zoological collections. Although the virus has been isolated from boids, colubrids and elapids, these groups are much less commonly affected.[217] Indeed, after one outbreak, a reticulated python was found to have the highest antibody titer of 22 snakes examined. This could indicate that nonviperids are carriers or hosts and viperids are aberrant very sensitive victims.[218] Virus transmission may be through the air or fomites, such as keepers, or cage cleaning utensils. Stress, such as in shipment, or ambient temperature fluctuations may activate latent infections.[219] Outbreaks often follow acquisitions of new animals with an ineffective quarantine.

Clinical signs following infection have been divided into three groups.[220] Those with acute infections, which make up the majority of cases, usually die within 3 to 10 weeks of exposure. Clinical signs can be minimal, such as anorexia or regurgitation, or no clinical signs may be evident and the snake is simply found dead. With longer infections, as respiratory signs develop, dyspnea and mucous discharge from the glottis may become evident, and serosanguineous fluid may be found in the cage. Neurologic signs such as ataxia, loss of equilibrium, head tremors, opisthotonus, and slow infrequent tongue flicking are less commonly observed just prior to death.[220,221,222] The third clinical picture includes those who chronically do poorly, who are often anorexic or hypophagic and may regurgitate. There may be lethargy, emaciaciation, decreased muscle tone, and heat seeking. Respiratory signs, as discussed, gaseous bowel distention, diarrhea, malodorous stools, and protozoan overgrowth may also be present.[220,222] The last group includes clinically healthy animals that may remain asymptomatic for up to 10 months while possibly shedding virus. Eventually most of these animals become chronic poor doers, although a few may recover.[220] Copperheads are thought to be one pit viper that may be resistant. Paramyxovirus causes a characteristic intersititial pneumonia if the snake does not die acutely. On necropsy one may find thickened pulmonary tissue and mucoid, or caseous, exudate, supporting secondary gram-negative infections (see Jacobson et al.[218] for histologic pathology).

Clinical suspicion of a paramyxovirus outbreak is raised with epidemic viperid die-offs, and a diagnosis can often be made with characteristic histopathology. Hemagglutination inhibition (HI) assay for antibody titers can help diagnose and evaluate the spread of paramyxovirus. Titers less than 1:20 are generally considered negative titers; higher antibody titers may represent active infection or previous exposure. A rising titer one month after the initial titer suggests active infection. Hemagglutination assays are available through veterinary schools at the University of Florida (contact Dr. Jacobson, test run once a month), the University of Tennessee (contact the virology laboratory), and Texas Veterinary Diagnostic laboratories. Supportive care of sick animals with antibiotics, fluids, nutritional support, and prefered temperatures is recommended, but many animals will die regardless of care. Isolation of affected animals, cagemates, or areas should continue for at least 3 months after the last death.[220] If quarantined animals are healthy and have negative titers after isolation, they are assumed to present little risk to other reptiles. Paramyxovirus is highly contagious (see quarantine section in chapter 1 for recommendations). Ethical individuals involved with outbreaks should advise colleagues interested in sending or recieving snakes from them of their current situation (see quarantine for more information). Killed vaccines produced a variable transient antibody response in western diamondback rattlesnkes. Modified live vaccine induced disease. Neither vaccine is currently in use.[219,223] For good reviews of paramyxovirus see Lloyd and Flanagan,[220] Flanagan, [222] or Cranfield and Graczyk.[223]

Cryptosporidiosis

Cryptosporidium serpentis is a coccidian parasite that can cause severe hypertrophic gastritis in snakes. Case reports have included boids (especially boa constrictors), elapids (especially Australian elapids), colubrids (especially rat and corn snakes, *Elaphe*), and viperids (especially rattlesnakes, *Crotalus*). Scattered case reports have also indicated lizards including chameleons, lacertids, monitors, and an iguana as being susceptible. Clinical signs in snakes classically include anorexia, lethargy, a firm midbody swelling (the stomach), with weight loss and persistent or intermittent postprandial regurgitation.[224] Regurgitation is usually 1 to 4 days after eating. Disease typically strikes mature snakes. Brownstein et al.[225] originally described mucous cell hyperplasia, which replaced granular cells (the reptilian equivalent of combined chief and parietal cells). This may explain the disruption in normal digestive processes. Instead of being partially digested, regurgitated prey is mucus covered, putrified, and maladorous. As digestive function ceases, the snake slowly starves to death or opportunistic bacterial infection overwhelms it. Diagnosis can be difficult in snakes without gastric thickening. Oocysts can be detected in mucus on regurgitated prey, stomach washes, aspirates, or fecals. Unfortunately, fecal direct smears and floats are often negative, in part because the small clear oocysts are easily overlooked or lightly shed. *Crypotosporidium*, or hidden sporocyst, was indeed well named, albiet for other reasons. Special stains (acid-fast, periodic acid–Schiff, and Giemsa) of heat-fixed slides are needed to identify cryptosporidia. A helpful hint is that cryptosporidia fail to stain with iodine but do stain with New Methylene Blue.[226,227] Barium studies may reveal pronounced gastric folds or gastric lumen narrowing.[228,229] Infections can also be detected in biopsy specimens from endoscopy, laparatomy, or even necropsy. Direct immunofluorescence with the Meriflour florescent antibody provides a much more sensitive test if one has a fluorescence microscope.[230]

There is no effective treatment. Infected snakes with chronic wasting and postprandial regurgitation over several weeks are best euthanized.[231] Subclinical snakes carrying cryptosporidia are an enigma in that they remain healthy.[230] Perhaps the cryptosporidia in these animals are an avirulent species from prey.[230] However, rodents do not become infected with *Cryptosporidium serpentis*, so they seem an unlikely source of disease.[224] Furthermore, there is no evidence that *C. serpentis* can infect mammals, but appropriate zoonotic precautions are still advisable.[230] This disease is a serious concern to large collections because, in addition to being difficult to detect and impossible to treat, oocysts survive well in the environment. Effective disinfectants (10% formal saline, 5% ammonia, undiluted commercial bleach) are extremely noxious and should not be used around animals.[227] Other common disinfectantants are not effective, except for hydrogen peroxide. Soaking for 10 minutes in hydrogen peroxide will kill oocyts even in the presence of organic matter.[231] Suspected cases should be strictly isolated and regurgitated material promptly, but carefully, disposed of. Disposable gloves and separate handling equipment are needed. Drying may decrease infectivity of oocysts.

Egg retention

Dystocia is common in colubrids and less common in pythons (recall that boas are live bearers) (figure 62). Many factors can lead to dystocia, such as lack of a nest box, a soiled nest box or presence of other snakes keeping the female out of the nest box, improper temperature gradients, too much handling or palpating, disturbance of the female's cage, immaturity (colubrids are best not bred before the second or third year), poor physical condition (such as lack of exercise or illness), dehydration, oviductal disease (rupture, torsion, prolapse, adhesions, infection), anomalous eggs (fused, swollen, misshapen, roughened, or infected eggs), or masses impinging on the oviduct (fecoliths, renal masses, or uroliths). It is crucial that gravid females have access to a nest box, a thermogradiant with basking area, and be minimally disturbed. Females shed 3 to 14 days (typically 7 to 10 days) prior to oviposition.[232] This is a good reference point for determining egg retention. Most females lay en masse overnight; rarely ovipositon may be strung out over several days, but this is certainly not typical. Therefore, a second indication of possible egg retention is that the female retains eggs more than 1 to 2 weeks after the first part of the clutch is laid. Clinical assessment is important, if the female is straining or not doing well than earlier intervention is indicated. It is always preferable for the female to lay on her own.

Initial assessment should include a good history and physical examination. Further work-up may include radiographs, ultrasonography, a complete blood count, or a plasma chemistry panel. Be certain the female is set up correctly; shallow lukewarm water soaks for 15 to 20 minutes may help.[233] If eggs are near the cloaca, gentle digital pressure, caudodorsally, may ease an egg or two out. It may be good to give the female another day if the remaining eggs are not easily manipulated. If resistance is felt, do not force the egg, or oviductal or mesenteric tearing may result. The egg may feel as if it is progressing caudally only to be tearing the oviductal mesentery. Dilating the cloaca of the anesthetized female may assist in extracting an egg through the oviductal opening (be sure it is not a tear). If the oviductal opening is not visible, a moist Q-tip may aid in finding and guiding it over the egg. If the eggs are retained high, they are unlikely to be milked to the cloaca. Pharmacologic intervention with oxytocin has generally been unrewarding but occasionally works.[234] Arginine vasotocin is a more natural and effective hormone than oxytocin for snakes, but high cost, short shelf life after reconstitution, and the need for experimental drug licensure to use it limit its usefulness.

Percutaneous or percloacal ovocentesis may collapse one or more eggs enough to allow natural delivery overnight.[233] To do this, stabilize the egg against the lateral body wall, and disinfect the skin. Using a 20- to 22-gauge needle and 6- to 12-cc syringe, one can often aspirate a few milliliters of yolk. If the yolk has solidified, aspiration is not feasible.

If these methods fail, salpingectomy is indicted. See Millichamp et al. [234] or Brown and Martin[235] for good reviews of surgical egg removal in snakes.The preferred site is the second or third scale rows from the ventrum, on the lateral body wall. The thin oviductal tissue is extremely difficult to suture. Advise the owner that recurrence of dystocia is likely in the future. However, the other oviduct may still be able to deliver a smaller clutch.

6

Caimans

The spectacled caiman (*Caiman crocodilus*) is a popular animal among reptile enthusiasts. It is easy to understand their appeal; hatchlings are widely available and make truly fascinating pets. Unfortunately, if fed and housed properly, they can grow a foot per year for the first few years and can rapidly outgrow their accommodations. Most crocodilians are severely endangered (some are close to extinction); however, spectacled caimans are not. Zoos often focus on more endangered crocodilians and thus have little space available to house unwanted spectacled caimans. Within a few years, the fascinating pet grows into a problem that nobody, including the owner, wants. They cannot even be given away. Some elect euthanasia at this point, but most caimans die from inadequate care well before they become big enough to become a problem. For these reasons, the author actively discourages individuals and pet stores from purchasing caimans. Nevertheless, they should still be cared for properly, and the veterinarian with an interest in reptiles occasionally sees them. Be forewarned: caimans are capable of serious bites. A quick grasp behind the head and over the pelvis secures smaller caimans. Placing a cloth over the head often makes capture easier. Larger caimens require several persons or chemical restraint (see chapter 7 on anesthesia).

Caiman Care

Temperature

Almost all crocodilians are tropical or at least semitropical reptiles; therefore they need a warm environment. Water temperature should be 24 to 28°C (75 to 82°F) at all times. Fully submersible aquarium heaters work admirably for this (see the section on aquatic turtle care in chapter 2). At temperatures below 25°C (77°F) appetite is decreased and below 20°C (68°F) caimans will not eat.[236] On many large crocodile farms, in temperate climates, the mortality rate is much higher in the colder winter months.[237]

Wild crocodilians rely on basking to warm their bodies; naturally radiant heat is also beneficial in captivity. Caimans need a "haul-out" area where they can get completely out of the water, dry off, and bask. A flat rock, driftwood just above the water level supported by bricks, or dry land section with a 75- to 100-watt incandescent bulb with reflector creates a basking area for small caimans. The light should be left on for 12 to 14 hours per day. The air temperature should drop to a low of 24˚C (75˚F) at night and gradually warm to 29 to 32˚C (85 or 90˚F) during the day. Ultraviolet lights are recommended (see chapter 1).

Housing

Clean water is important. Frequent full water changes are the best way to guarantee clean water. Large-capacity out-of-tank filters can be used, but water should still be changed regularly even if the water looks clean. Dechlorination of water is not necessary. See chapter 1 for more on water quality and its importance.

Aquariums make good cages, but keep in mind that caimans grow rapidly, so start with as large an aquarium as possible. Galvanized watering troughs, plastic wading pools, koi ponds (remove the koi first), or sealed refrigerator liners also make good cages. Make sure the cages have secure-fitting lids, or the caiman will climb out. For ease of cleaning and to prevent gastrointestinal impaction, do not put gravel on the bottom. Cages with a half land section built into the aquarium and filled with gravel are difficult to clean and should be avoided. Remember, the simpler the cage, the easier it will be to keep clean and the healthier the caiman will be in the long run.

Feeding

Diet is another difficult area. In the wild llanos of central Venezuela, spectacled caimans feed mainly on fish during the dry season, mammals from the late dry season to the early wet season, and snails and crabs during the rainy season.[238] Smaller caiman eat fish, snails, crabs, and insects (particularly giant water bugs [Belostomids] and aquatic and terrestrial beetles), whereas larger caimans eat fish, mammals, reptiles, birds, crabs, snails, and amphibians. In general, there is a shift to larger prey items and less insects as the caimans grow. In captivity it is important to feed as much variety as possible. Juvenile caimans should eat dusted insects of all types (crickets, waxworms, mealworms, grasshoppers, moths, beetles, flies, etc.), earthworms, fish (chopped or whole goldfish, smelt, trout, catfish, herring, mackerel, and others), chopped or whole mice and other rodents, and whole shrimp (not shelled). As caimans grow, larger prey items such as fish, rats, other rodents (guinea pigs, nutria), rabbits, chickens (pluck larger feathers), pigeons, and pigs can be provided. Whole mice are nutritionally balanced and should provide the bulk of the diet. Small amounts of meat products, such as chicken necks, gizzards, livers, and horsemeat, can be offered periodically but are not a balanced diet by themselves and may be a source of *Salmonella*. Avoid strips of raw beef or hamburger. Sole reliance on any one food item is not healthy, except perhaps for whole rodents. All fish diets, especially if frozen, can lead to steatitis or vitamin B deficiency. If caimans are offered food from a dish placed on the haul-out area, they eventually will eat anything placed in the dish with alacrity. Hatchlings should be fed three to five times per week and larger caimans two to three times per week. Remember, variety is the key to a healthy diet. If a balanced diet is fed, heavy vitamin and mineral supplementation is probably not needed (with the exception of commercial farming operations).

Several problems can be encountered with feeding frozen fish exclusively. Steatitis (fat inflammation) followed by steatosis (fat cell degeneration with sparse inflammatory reaction) is a common cause of death in crocodilians fed large amounts of frozen fish, such as mackerel or smelt,[241] or fish exclusively, especially rancid fish.[242] Besides not eating, there are few clinical signs, as most affected animals appear grossly normal.[242] Occasionally, in severe cases, necrotic brown ulcers may be seen in the mouth, cloaca, or skin, or palpable indurated fatty tissue may be present.[10,241] Upon necropsy, firm yellow-brown masses are distributed in fat tissue throughout the body.[242] These areas produce an orange fluorescence with ultraviolet light.[241] High levels of polyunsaturated fatty acids are typical for marine and coldwater fish species.[243] Polyunsaturation enhances peroxidation of these oils, which consumes vitamin E stores in the fish. Ceroid is produced as a metabolite and accumulates in the reptile as the focus for steatitis. Oxidized or rancid fats also increase vitamin E requirements for the fish eater.[243] Fish should be supplemented with 20 IU of vitamin E per day and sick animals should be supplemented with 100 IU of vitamin E per day.[244] Oxidation can be decreased by using good quality fish (i.e., fish without breaks in the skin, ruptured viscera, freezer burn, or spoilage), tightly wrapping frozen fish, and minimizing freezer storage time.[12,243] Once again, feeding a balanced diet will prevent the problem altogether.

All-fish diets can also lead to thiamine deficiencies because of thiaminases found in many fish. Red donkey meat also induced thiamine deficiencies in farmed saltwater crocodile hatchlings in Australia.[245] Clinical signs include anorexia, emaciation, lethargy, incoordination, front limb paralysis, open jaws, loss of righting reflex, and drowning or death.[10,244,245] Recovery was rapid, within a day or two, after two 30-mg thiamine hydrochloride injections.[245] Interestingly, some cases, which could not be treated for up to a week, showed no progression of nervous signs and still recovered rapidly following thiamine injections.[245] Frye[12] recommends 25 mg/kg thiamine HCl q 24 hr for three to seven treatments. To prevent thiamine deficiencies one can supplement food with brewer's yeast capsules or thiamine HCl tablets and feed a wider variety of foods.

Diseases of Caimans

Metabolic bone disease

The most common problems in caimans result from improper husbandry. Metabolic bone disease (MBD) is a frequent fate of caimans fed beef strips, insects, and chicken parts without whole animals, such as mice or fish, in their diet. Young crocodilians grow at fantastic rates which predisposes them to metabolic bone disease. Webb and colleagues[239] found that young saltwater crocodiles selected a calcium-rich diet (about 7 parts Ca to 1 part P), whereas larger, slower growing crocodiles selected a diet with 1.8 parts Ca to 1 part P (see feeding insectivorus reptiles and amphibians in chapter 4 for more detail). Symptoms of MBD may include anorexia, lethargy, weakness, difficulty walking, kyphoscoliosis, shortening of the axial skeleton, deformed or rubbery jaws, fibrous osteodystrophy of the long bones, tooth loss, or teeth jutting from the mouth at oblique angles.[10,240] Diagnosis and treatment are similar to those for green iguanas. Provision of whole animal diets (i.e., with bones) prevents the problem altogether.

Blood sampling is fairly easy in small crocodilians as they are bled from the tail vein in the same manner as lizards. In large crocodilians the ventral coccygeal vein is inaccessible without spinal needles. Larger crocodilians are best bled from a postoccipital venous sinus dorsal to the spinal cord.[12,240] Contamination with cerebrospinal fluid and pithing of the spinal cord can be problematic. The postoccipital venous sinus is on midline just caudal to the occiput (roughly 1.5 cm in a large crocodilian).

Hypoglycemic shock

Hypoglycemic shock has been reported in crocodilians secondary to stress such as cold, overcrowding, or struggle with capture.[246] Symptoms include mydriasis (or miosis if agitated), tremors, star gazing (snout pointing upward), torpor, and a slow to absent righting reflex.

Treatment consists of stomach tubing with glucose at 3 g/kg or 2 g of table sugar dissolved in 12 ml of water per kilogram of body weight.[244]

Parasitic infections

Parasitic infections, particularly coccidiosis and pentastomiasis, are common in farm situations with wild-caught animals. Coccidiosis causes enteritis of varying severity in a variety of crocodilians, especially young animals in crowded situations.[240,247] Pentastomids are a common worldwide farm problem; *Sebekia oxycephala* has been incriminated in American alligators.[248] Adult pentastomids migrate into the lungs and can cause severe, secondary, bacterial, exudative pneumonias. Nymphal pentastomids are found in other body tissues such as the liver. Mortality can be high, particularly among hatchlings with heavy exposure. Fish are thought to be the intermediate host. Freezing mosquito fish (*Gambusia affinis*) at negative 10°C (14°F) for 72 hours was found to kill *Sebekia* larvae.[248]

Visceral gout

Visceral gout is a less common problem in crocodilians but does crop up, typically if they are being fed heavily for growth. White precipitates are found around enlarged kidneys and sometimes around the heart, joints, or other coelomic organs.[237] Jacobson[240] mentioned suspected gout cases with front limb paralysis, followed by rear limb paralysis and death, if feeding continued. If symptomatic cases were fasted for a week, the alligators quickly recovered.

Pox Virus

Occasionally pox virus is seen and causes raised, gray-white, circular, small (1 to 6 mm) multifocal plaques on the skin, especially on the head (figure 63). Pox virus outbreaks have also been reported in farmed 1- to 2-year-old Nile crocodiles[249,250] and are fairly common in imported hatchling caimans. Pox infections generally run their course in about a month. Most individual caimans with good captive care survive; however, in one outbreak in Africa, farm fatality was more than 25%.[250] Pox lesions can damage crocodile skin destined for the leather trade. Horner[249] described a simple autogenous vaccine that resulted in faster healing with less skin damage.

Infections

Crocodilians are also susceptible to a wide variety of deep and superficial fungal infections.[237,240] Most fungal infections are associated with inadequate environmental temperatures. Deep mycoses typically affect the lungs. Hepatic or intestinal infection is also possible.[237] Superficial mycotic infections create pale gelatinous areas on the head, belly, and tail with or without skin ulceration or erythema.[10,237]

Opportunistic infections are common under adverse environmental conditions with a variety of bacteria. Frequently incriminated bacteria include *Aeromonas hydrophila*, *Pasturella multocida*, *Staphylococcus aureus*, *Salmonella,* and other gram-negative pathogens. Alligators with *Aeromonas hydrophila* skin lesions exhibited heterophilia (heterophils constituted 73% of the differential count, about 5900/μl, compared with 37%, or about 2000/μl, for normal alligators).[251] Heterophils returned to normal 1 to 2 weeks after the alligators responded adequately to the infection or the lesions were treated with antibiotics.[251] Symptoms of pneumonia include coughing, sneezing, and nasal discharge. Multiple pathogens (bacterial, fungal, parasitic) should be considered with pneumonias. Symptoms of septicemia include subcutaneous edema, ulceration, and erythema of skin on the belly and tail.

For Further Reading

For more information on crocodilian diseases see Jacobson,[240] Buenviaj et al.,[237] Ladds et al.,[247] and Youngprapakorn et al.[10] For detailed natural history and management information, see Ross,[252] Webb et al.,[253] and Bolton.[236]

7

Anesthesia of Reptiles

General Considerations

Veterinarians less experienced in reptilian anesthesia are understandably apprehensive about it, because of the variety of anesthetics from which to choose and inexperience in using most of them on reptiles. Reptilian anesthesia can be done in a safe, consistent manner with the same degree of confidence one has anesthetizing other species. A basic review of reptile physiology is indicated before discussing specific anesthetics.

Reptiles are ectotherms, or extrinsically temperature dependent. Therefore, their body temperature, metabolism, heart rate, and response to anesthetics depend on ambient temperature. Reptiles must be kept warm before, during, and after anesthesia so that their metabolism remains consistent and their response to anesthesia predictable. In general, most reptiles do best when kept between 24 and 30°C (75 and 86°F). A space heater is useful for keeping a room within these temperatures so that patients can be acclimated to this temperature before and during induction of anesthesia and returned to it when well recovered. During anesthesia and until moderately recovered, ambient temperatures of 24 to 27°C (75 to 80°F) are practical for most veterinary facilities and still within the preferred body temperature range of most reptiles. Anesthetic induction and recovery times with halothane were increased with temperatures above or below 24 to 30°C (75 to 86°F).[254] Use of a heating pad, circulating water blanket, or heated surgical table will keep reptiles warm during surgery.

Hypothermia or cold narcosis is not, under any circumstances, recommended. Hypothermia lowers the reptile's metabolism enough that it responds slowly to painful stimuli, yet nerve conduction is still present.[255,256] There is little or no evidence that it provides analgesia; the reptile simply can no longer react to the painful stimulus.[12,255] In addition, chilling decreases reptilian immune responses and may predispose the patient to opportunistic infections. More humane methods of anesthesia should be employed.

Reptiles may have a renal portal system, which means blood draining from the tail and pelvic limbs passes through a capillary bed in the kidneys before returning to the vena cava for systemic circulation. Theoretically, this could be significant for drugs that are nephrotoxic or excreted through the kidneys. A study of two different drugs injected in the cranial or caudal half of red-eared sliders demonstrated pharmacokinetic differences in one drug, but not enough to be clinically significant.[257] Rather than concentrate on the potential for kidney excretion, it is common practice to inject drugs in the cranial half of the reptiles body, if feasible.

Another important consideration before anesthesia is the health status of the reptile. A thorough physical examination and any indicated blood work should precede anesthesia. Emaciated, dehydrated, or severely ill reptiles are poor anesthetic risks. If at all possible, avoid anesthesia until the patient is more stable.

Common Anesthetics

Several anesthetics are in common usage. Injectable anesthetics include ketamine HCl, tiletamine HCl and zolazepam HCl, lidocaine, and propofol. For more invasive surgeries, gas anesthesia with isoflurane is preferred.

Ketamine is useful for mild chemical restraint but its analgesic properties are questionable. Ketamine is generally used for minor procedures such as lancing abscesses or assisting with venipuncture. When a true surgical plane of anesthesia is required, ketamine is useful as a preanesthetic for gas anesthesia. See the anesthetic section of chapter 8 for dose ranges. Note that large dose ranges are listed because larger reptiles with slower metabolisms will require lower mg/kg dosages than smaller reptiles that have higher metabolic rates.[258,259] The lower end of these dosages will produce tranquilization and the higher end deeper sedation and perhaps apnea. Some movement of the patient is possible even at higher dosages. If necessary, smaller additional dosages can be given at 30-minute intervals in 10-mg/kg increments.[260,261] Higher dosages of ketamine can be used, with ventilatory support, but it is safer to use inhalation anesthesia. Sedation after ketamine injection occurs within 15 to 30 minutes and immobilization lasts for up to 20 minutes. Recovery usually takes 3 to 4 hours, although it can take hours to days, depending on the dosage and animal. Higher doses will increase recovery time. Lizards usually recover faster than snakes, and crocodilians and turtles take even longer.[262] As ketamine is excreted through the kidneys, it should not be used in reptiles with suspected kidney impairment or severe dehydration.[12,263,264]

A newer related anesthetic, tiletamine HCl and zolazepam HCl (Telazol, AH Robbins, Richmond, VA), also works well in reptiles. Telazol is two to three times more potent than ketamine, facilitating smaller volumes and more rapid onset. Telazol produces smoother sedation with more muscle relaxation than ketamine. In iguanas the onset of action is within 10 to 15 minutes, with about a half-hour duration of immobilization. See the anesthetic section of chapter 8 for dosages. After reconstitution it can be refrigerated and used for up to 1 month. As with ketamine, severe respiratory depression is possible, especially at higher dosages, which can be overcome with intermittent positive pressure ventilation (IPPV) until the patient begins spontaneously breathing again.

Local anesthesia with 0.5% to 2% lidocaine works very well for minor surgical procedures such as biopsies, tail or digit amputations, or minor wound repair. Lidocaine is infiltrated into or just proximal to the target tissue. Two percent lidocaine can be diluted with an equal volume of 0.9% saline. For patients that are difficult to restrain, a sedative dose of ketamine or telazol is advised.

Another new anesthetic is the ultrashort-acting hypnotic propofol.[263,264] Propofol has the advantages of rapid onset (within 1 to 5 minutes) and rapid smooth recovery (within 25 to 40 minutes). Surgical anesthesia lasts 15 to 25 minutes, making this an excellent anesthetic for short procedures or induction. The key disadvantage is intravenous administration, which can be difficult in snakes, chelonians, and crocodilians but is relatively easy through the ventral coccygeal vein in lizards (see venipuncture in the section Basic Medical Techniques for Green Iguanas in chapter 3). In chelonians the jugular vein and dorsal tail vein are the easiest sites for administration. An intravenous catheter simplifies usage but again is technically difficult to establish (see Mader[266] for a review). Intraosseous administration is another option.[333] Propofol is a white, opaque liquid that passes easily through needles as small as 27 gauge. It is not painful with injection and perivascular injection does not cause problems. See Divers[265] and Bennett et al.[333] for more information.

For most major invasive surgeries, gas anesthesia is indicated. Premedication with atropine (0.01 to 0.04 mg/kg SC or IM) or glycopyrrolate (0.01 mg/kg SC or IM) is recommended to reduce oral and upper respiratory tract secretions and to prevent bradycardia.[12,13,260] Small endotracheal tubes in tiny patients are especially prone to blockage by upper respiratory tract secretions. The only volatile anesthetic the author has used in reptiles is isoflurane, although many others also recommend halothane. Most snakes can be intubated easily but other reptiles need to be sedated first with injectable anesthetics, mask induced, or placed in an anesthetic chamber. Reptiles can undergo prolonged apnea, so masking down can take anywhere from minutes to half an hour and anesthetic chambers often take longer. Chelonians can be especially difficult to induce in this manner because they are capable of long periods of apnea. Intermittent positive-pressure ventilation can overcome apnea but the reptile has to be intubated first. Once the reptile loses its righting reflex, it can be intubated.

In reptiles the glottis is open only during inhalation and remains closed otherwise (the reverse of the situation in mammals). The glottis is located just caudal to the base of the tongue in all species except crocodilians. Crocodilians have a muscular valve (the basihyal valve) arising from the ventral floor of the mouth that seals the glottis off from the oral cavity so that they can feed underwater. Once they are preanesthetized, a tongue depressor or laryngoscope can depress the basihyal valve ventrally to expose the glottis. The glottis is easiest to visualize in snakes. The large fleshy tongue of certain lizards and chelonians makes glottal visualization more difficult. The glottis can be pushed anteriorly and more easily visualized by craniodorsal laryngeal elevation from under the throat. It is advisable to use a speculum in large chelonians, lizards, and crocodilians to prevent accidental bites.

Endotracheal tubes can be fashioned from tom cat catheters for very small patients or red rubber feeding tubes cut to size. Cole tubes also work well. Cuffed infant endotracheal tubes can be used for very large reptiles. Crocodilians and chelonians have complete tracheal rings, hence their tracheas are less expandable, so take care not to overinflate the endotracheal tube cuff. After locating the glottis, wait until it opens, or gently force the endotracheal tube through the glottal opening. When the tube is in place it should be taped to either jaw with white adhesive tape (otherwise it is sure to come out). In some chelonians, the trachea bifurcates a short distance down the neck. Care must be taken not to pass an endotracheal tube too caudally and inadvertently cannulate only one primary bronchus.[263]

Nonrebreathing circuits are recommended for reptiles under 10 kg.[262] Oxygen flow is set at 300 to 500 ml/kg/min. Induction with halothane should be at 3%, isoflurane at 3% to 5%, and maintenance with halothane at 1.5% to 2%, isoflurane at 1% to 2%.[258,259] Generally, gas anesthesia is not as smooth in reptiles as in other animals, so it is wise to restrain the reptile securely. Frequently the patient will appear to be at a surgical plane of anesthesia and then start struggling and appear wide awake with little warning. In part this is because it is preferable to keep reptiles at a light surgical plane of anesthesia and recovery from isoflurane is rapid. Also, depth of anesthesia is more difficult to assess in reptiles and reptiles are capable of long periods of apnea, which reduces anesthetic gas exchange.

Monitoring Anethesia

Depth of anesthesia can be monitored by pinching the tail or cloaca of snakes or the nail bed, digits, or cloaca of other species. One of the first reflexes lost is the ability of the reptile to right itself.[263] Reflexes are lost cranially to caudally and recovered in the opposite direction.[263] Respiration slows down considerably from 10 to 20 breaths per minute in a snake to 2 to 4 breaths per minute as anesthesia progresses.[262] At this point, IPPV is required at 2 to 4 breaths per minute.[259,260] Be careful not to overinflate the lungs and rupture the fragile air sacs. Watch the patient while bagging to ascertain the extent of air sac expansion. Mechanical ventilation is not recommended for small reptiles.[266] At deeper levels of anesthesia chelonians' limbs and head will hang limply out of their shell (loss of head withdrawal reflex). Snakes should retract their tongue if it is gently withdrawn from its sheath at a surgical plane of anesthesia but lose this reflex with excessive depth of anesthetia.[267] The corneal reflex is lost in the deepest stage of anesthesia in lizards and chelonians[254,262] but should be present at a surgical plane of anesthesia.[263] Snakes lack eyelids and therefore have no corneal reflex.

Recovery from isoflurane depends on the length of anesthesia. IPPV should continue with room air until the patient is breathing well on its own (usually less than an hour). Keep a close eye on the patient during recovery; periodically pinching a toe or tail seems to stimulate respiration and speed recovery. Lawton[264] recommends doxapram HCl (Dopram-V, 20 mg/ml, Fort Dodge) at 0.25 ml/kg IV to stimulate spontaneous respiration and decrease postoperative observation. Mader[268] suggests that the slow recovery of reptiles may be due to tissue oxygen saturation. Reptiles, unlike mammals, regulate their respiratory rate through balance of oxygen partial pressure and body temperature. Bagging with oxygen may actually inhibit the return to spontaneous respiration.[268]

The three-chambered reptilian heart does not produce readily auscultable sounds, making stethoscopy difficult.[267] Therefore a two- to four-lead electrocardiogram (EKG) is more useful for monitoring heart rate and anesthetic depth. Once snakes lose their righting reflex, the heart can be visualized as it beats against the ventral scales, usually about one-third of the total body length from the head. Small-gauge needles can be placed through skin and muscle anterior and posterior to the heart and then attached to the EKG clips. The heart in iguanids lies between the shoulders (not caudal to the front legs); therefore this author prefers to place EKG leads (again attached to needles through skin and muscle) along the left neck and along the body wall posterior to the right humeri. In monitors the heart is situated one-third to one-half the distance between the front and rear limbs, thus traditional EKG placement is indicated. Heart rate should be kept close to the rate present at the start of anesthesia. A decrease in heart rate necessitates a decrease in anesthetic concentration, but remember that heart rate is also temperature dependent.

Doppler ultrasonic flow detectors are useful on limbs or the head of reptiles to pick up a pulse. Pulse oximetry is just starting to be used in reptiles and offers much promise for monitoring both pulse and oxygenation.[268] Rectal or esophageal probes are more reliable than trying to keep a probe on the tongue. With an esophageal probe, the diodes should be placed adjacent to the internal carotids–jugular vein complex. In patients in which this is not feasible, the probe can be inserted rectally (with disposable plastic sheaths) and the diodes directed dorsally to read the caudal aorta and renal arteries.[268] The latter technique works quite well in iguanas.

Keep the patient warm during surgery with a circulating water blanket and have it recover on a towel placed over a heating pad set on low. Intermittent positive pressure ventilation should continue with room air postoperatively until the patient is spontaneously respiring (usually less than an hour). Pinching toes will encourage spontaneous respiration. Be sure to monitor the patient closely until respiration is consistent.

Keep in mind that a wide spectrum of anesthetics have been used in reptiles, yet one can accomplish most procedures with just the few mentioned choices. Remember to maintain temperatures and avoid anesthesia in poor anesthetic candidates. Monitor the patient closely during and after anesthesia, until it is fully recovered and breathing regularly and spontaneously. Use the lower end of the anesthetic dosages until you have an idea of their effect, and remember that larger patients require a smaller mg/kg dosage than smaller patients. Reptile anesthesia generally does not proceed as smoothly as anesthesia in other animals, but do not let this frustrate you. Also keep in mind that, as more is learned, much of what is now recommended may change.

For Further Reading

For more extensive reviews of reptilian anesthesia the reader is referred to Bennett,[263,269] Frye,[12] Lawton,[264] or Schumacher.[270]

8

Reptile Formulary

General Guidelines

Drug use in reptiles and amphibians has traditionally been heavily empirical. Most studies on the use of antibiotics in reptiles present preliminary results derived from short antibiotic trials. Little is known about long-term drug accumulation, yet the slow metabolism of reptiles often dictates long-term drug usage. For instance, the author typically treats bacterial infections for a minimum of 3 weeks. With so little known it behooves the practitioner to observe some basic guidelines.

1. Use antibiotics only when there is a strong likelihood of bacterial infection; avoid antibiotic usage to placate clients.[271] Instead of relying on antibiotics to treat an unknown disease, utilize diagnostics to find out what the problem is.[271]

2. Start treatment as early as possible after having taken samples for bacterial culture and sensitivity.[271] The presence of multiple bacteria, with multiple antibiotic resistance, is the norm for infections in reptiles.[271] Anaerobic infections are quite common,[272] yet the most frequently used antibiotics in reptiles, fluoroquinolones and aminoglycosides, are relatively useless for anaerobes. Sensitivity testing allows one to select the right antibiotic well before a clinical response is apparent. Avoid frequent switching of antibiotics.

3. Select bactericidal antibiotics over bacteriostatic antibiotics[13] unless sensitivity testing dictates otherwise. The

author prefers to use antibiotics with some reptilian pharmacokinetic data.

4. Some reptiles have a renal portal system with valves that allow blood to be shunted through or around the kidneys. Drugs injected in the hind region of reptiles could circulate through the kidneys before reaching the systemic circulation or bypass the kidneys altogether. Theoretically, this could reduce therapeutic levels of drugs excreted through the kidneys or increase the nephrotoxicicity of certain drugs. One study[273] supports the presence of a renal portal system in red-eared sliders. Holz and colleagues found that forelimb versus hindlimb injection had no significant effect on gentamicin, a drug excreted through glomerular filtration. In contrast, differences were found for carbenicillin, a drug excreted by glomerular filtration and tubular secretion. Turtles injected with carbenicillin in the rear limbs had significantly lower blood levels of carbenicillin for the first 12 hours after injection than those injected in the forelimbs. Even though the differences were statistically significant, the minimal inhibitory concentrations (MICs) from both sites were high enough to be effective for most organisms treated with carbenicillin, so that the therapeutic effect would be similar for either site.[273] This study indicates that the renal portal system may have effects on drugs excreted through tubular secretion, the significance of which is unknown. Therefore, until more is known, it is best to give drugs excreted through the kidneys in the front half of reptiles, rather than focusing on the nephrotoxic or tubular secretion potential.[274]

5. When calculating drug doses for chelonians, do not adjust for shell weight because the shell is likely to be metabolically active.[275]

6. Reptiles are ectothermic and pharmacokinetics of drugs are thus heavily influenced by ambient temperature. Numerous studies[276–279] have shown that drug clearance is slower at lower environmental temperatures (because of lower metabolic rate), which can lead to drug accumulation and potential toxicity. It is crucially important that reptiles be acclimated and maintained within their preferred optimum temperature zone (POTZ) while treated with potentially nephrotoxic drugs.[279] In addition, one study found the MICs for some bacterial pathogens were lower at 37°C (98.6°F) than at 25°C (77°F).[278] Therefore, increased temperature may not only increase immune system activity but also enhance antibiotic effectiveness. Thus, try to select temperatures within the POTZ that reasonably coincide with temperatures from pharmacokinetic studies.[280] The POTZ for many species is from 24 to 30°C (75 to 85°F), but sick reptiles do better between 27 and 32°C (80 and 90°F). In the veterinary hospital it is best to dedicate a room for reptiles heated to the desired temperature. Alternatives are incubators or heating pads kept at the desired temperature. Be aware that temperatures over 38°C (100°F) are rapidly lethal for many reptiles. Debilitated reptiles are sometimes too weak to move from a heat source. Monitor temperatures and animals closely to avoid overheating, dehydration, or death. Unfortunately, temperature affects not only metabolic rate but also blood and tissue pH (pH drops with increasing temperature), which in turn affects antibiotic bioavailability and toxicity.[281] This may explain the increased gentamicin nephrotoxicity at higher temperatures that Hodge[277] observed in water snakes,[281] or perhaps it is a reflection of increased susceptibility to toxicity of more metabolically active cells.

7. All drug use in reptiles and amphibians is extra-label. The great diversity of species and ecology is likely to ensure that there will be major differences between different reptiles and amphibians. What applies to one species may not prove true in another species. Nonetheless, one must frequently extrapolate known reptilian pharmacokinetics from one species to another. Use potentially toxic drugs with extreme caution and avoid long-term usage. Preliminary results indicate that aminoglycosides and enrofloxacin may accumulate in a stepwise fashion over time.

Additional Guidelines for Specific Drugs

Aminoglycosides

Aminoglycosides function poorly in abscesses, in the presence of exudates, under conditions of low oxygen availability such as hypoxic tissue, and against anaerobes. Two aminoglycosides have been investigated in reptiles, gentamicin and amikacin, both of which enjoy little antibiotic resistance (less than 10% in one study).[282] Of the two, gentamicin is widely assumed to have a much narrower therapeutic index. Gentamicin-induced nephrotoxicity has been documented in snakes.[283,284] The likelihood of nephrotoxicity can be reduced by avoiding aminoglycoside usage in dehydrated patients, maintaining good hydration during treatment, and monitoring plasma uric acids before, during, and 2 weeks after the last treatment. Unfortunately, plasma uric acid levels are an insensitive indicator of renal disease, as two-thirds of functional renal mass must be lost before blood levels become elevated.[285] Elevated plasma uric acid levels should be cause for concern.[286,287] Some snakes and carnivorous lizards have elevated uric acid levels for several days postprandially and it might be advantageous to minimize feeding if clinical conditions permit this.[286] It is important to ensure adequate hydration by providing suitable access to water, and consider 15 to 25 ml/kg of fluids via gavage, subcutaneously, or epi- or intracoelomically.[287,288] Although additional fluids may not be required, they certainly would do no harm. In addition, pay attention to ambient temperatures and match those closely to the temperatures of known pharmacokinetic trials. As aminoglycosides appear to accumulate in a stepwise fashion over time, therapy beyond 2 weeks is particularly worrisome.[289] Johnson et al.[285] recommended only a single dose of amikacin because of concern about nephrotoxicity. Transcutaneous absorption of aminoglycosides is possible in amphibians, but erratic serum levels and toxicity contraindicate this method of delivery.[290] Aminoglycosides should not be used in conjunction with loop diuretics such as furosemide, and combination with carbenicillin, ticarcillin, or piperacillin is problematic (see below). Given the safety of other broad-spectrum antibiotics, aminoglycosides are not typically the author's first choice for reptiles.

Penicillins and cephalosporins

These drugs generally have broad-spectrum bactericidal activity against a variety of aerobic and anaerobic pathogens; unfortunately, they tend to be expensive (except for ampicillin). One study found 85% of reptilian aerobic bacterial isolates to be resistant to ampicillin; only 35% were resistant to carbenicillin.[282] Ceftazidime is apparently an excellent drug against *Pseudomonas*. Penicillins and cephalosporins have a much safer therapeutic index than the aminoglycosides and may be synergistic in combination with aminoglycosides. Combination therapy involves some inherent difficulties, such as potential inactivation of gentamicin by carbenicillin. They should not be mixed in a syringe and the dosages should be staggered. Jacobson[286] recommends starting carbenicillin 48 hours after aminoglycoside administration. Once reconstituted, many antibiotics have a shelf life of 72 hours if refrigerated, but they can be aliquoted and frozen for longer usage. Carbenicillin causes pain on injection.[281]

Chloramphenicol

The bacteriostatic nature of this drug makes it less useful in reptiles except for several anaerobes and *Salmonella* or unless the sensitivity pattern leaves no alternatives. Most *Pseudomonas* are resistant to it. Note that there is a wide variation in dosing intervals. One of nine water snakes (*Nerodia* spp.) developed greenish plasma after 9 days of chloramphenicol (CHPC) at 50 mg/kg SC q 72 hr and was anemic when the PCV was checked on day 18 of the study.[291] Focal indurations may develop at the injection site of CHPC preparations suspended in propylene glycol and benzyl alcohol.[286]

Fluoroquinolones

These drugs have good gram-negative aerobic activity as well as effectiveness against *Mycoplasma* and *Mycobacteria*. *Pseudomonas* and *Citrobacter* spp. require higher minimal inhibitory concentrations, which can be achieved by decreasing the dosing interval or increasing the dosage. Fluoroquinolones have a wide spectrum of safety and little bacterial resistance at this time. Ciprofloxacin can be suspended in distilled water and given via gavage, which is practical for large snakes. Enrofloxacin is irritating when given SC or IM; therefore injection sites should be varied. Skin necrosis and permanent skin discoloration has developed in snakes. Oral enrofloxacin, either from crushed suspended tablets or injectable form, produces good clinical results.

For Further Reading

For more in-depth discusssions of therapeutics see Klingenberg,[288] Jacobson,[292] and Mader.[287]

Table 1
Reptilian and Amphibian Drug Dosages

Antibiotics and Antifungal Dosages Based on Limited Pharmacokinetic Studies

Drug Dose/Route/Interval	Species, °C (°F)
Amikacin	
2.25 mg/kg IM q 72 hr	American alligator, *Alligator m. mississippiensis,* 22°C (72°F)[293]
5 mg/kg IM q 48 hr	Gopher tortoise, *Gopherus polyphemus*, 30°C (86°F)[279]
5 mg/kg IM initially, then 2.5 mg/kg q 72 hr	Gopher snake, *Pituophis melanoleucus* spp., 37°C (99°F)[278]
3.48 mg/kg IM once	Ball python, *Python regius*, 25°C (77°F) or 37°C (98.6°F)[285]
Ampicillin	
50 mg/kg IM q 12 hr	Hermann's tortoise, *Testudo hermanni*, 27°C (81°F)[294]
Carbenicillin	
400 mg/kg IM q 24 hr	Mangrove snake, *Boiga dendrophilia*, King snake, *Lampropeltus g. getulus*, Reticulated python, *Python reticulatus*, Rat snakes, *Elaphe* spp., 30°C (86°F)[295]
400 mg/kg IM q 48 hr	Mediterranean tortoises, *Testudo graeca*, *T. hermanni*, 30°C (86°F)[296]
Ciprofloxacin	
2.5 mg/kg PO q 48–72 hr	Reticulated pythons, *Python reticulatus*, 27°C (81°F)[297]
Cefoperazone	
100 mg/kg IM q 96 hr	False water cobras, *Hydrodynastes gigas,* 24°C (75°F)[334]
125 mg/kg IM q 24 hr	Black tegu, *Tupinambis teguixin,* 24°C (75°F)[335]
Ceftazidime	
20 mg/kg IM q 72 hr	Mangrove snake, *Boiga dendrophilia*, Boids (pythons and boas), Rat snake, *Elaphe obsoleta* spp., 30°C (86°F)[298]

continued

20 mg/kg IM or IV q 72 hr	Loggerhead sea turtles, *Caretta caretta*[299]

Chloramphenicol

40 mg/kg SC q 24 hr	Gopher snake, *Pituophis melanoleucus* spp., 29°C (84°F)[276]
50 mg/kg SC q 12 hr	Indigo, *Drymarchon* spp., Rat, *Elaphe* spp., King snakes, *Lampropeltis* spp., 24–28°C (75–82°F)[291]
50 mg/kg SC q 24 hr	Boa, *Boa constrictor*, Burmese python *Python molorus bivittatus*, Copperhead, cottonmouth, *Agkistrodon* spp., Hog-nose snake, *Heterodon* spp. 24–28°C (75–82°F)[291]
50 mg/kg SC q 48 hr	Rattlesnakes, *Crotalus* spp., 24–28°C (75–82°F)[291]
50 mg/kg SC q 72 hr	Water snakes, *Nerodia* spp., 24–28°C (75–82°F)[291]

Doxycycline

50 mg/kg IM (rear leg), then 25 mg/kg at 72 hr, then 25 mg/kg at 120 hr	Hermann's tortoise, *Testudo hermanni,* 27°C (81°F)[294]

Enrofloxacin

6.6 mg/kg IM q 24 hr or 11 mg/kg IM q 48 hr	Reticulated pythons, *Python reticulatus,* 27°C (81°F)[300]
10 mg/kg IM q 48 hr for *Pseudomonas*	Burmese pythons, *Python molurus bivittatus,* 30°C (86°F)[301]
10 mg/kg IM initially, then 5 mg/kg IM q 48 hr for other bacteria	Burmese pythons, *Python molurus bivittatus,* 30°C (86°F)[301]
5 mg/kg IM q 24–48 hr	Gopher tortoises, *Gopherus polyphemus,* 29–31°C (84–88°F)[302]
5 mg/kg IM q 12–24 hr	Star tortoises, *Geochelone elegans,* 26–30°C (79–86°F)[303]
10 mg/kg q 24 hr	Hermann's tortoise, *Testudo hermanni,* 27°C (81°F)[294]
5 mg/kg PO q 32 hr 5 mg/kg IM q 16 hr	Green iguana, *Iguana iguana*[304]
5 mg/kg IV q 36 hr	American alligator, *Alligator mississippiensis,* 27°C (81°F)[305]

Gentamicin

2.5 mg/kg IM q 72 hr	Gopher snake, *Pituophis melanoleucus* spp., 24°C (75°F)[276]
2.5 mg/kg IM initially, then 1.5 mg/kg q 96 hr	Blood python, *Python curtus,* 28–30°C (82–86°F)[306]
1.75 mg/kg IM q 72–96 hr	American alligator, *Alligator m. mississippiensis,* 22°C (72°F)[293]
6 mg/kg IM q 96–120 hr	Red-eared slider, *Chrysemys scripta elegans,* 23–25 °C (73–77 °F)[307]
3 mg/kg IM q 24 hr	Leopard frog, *Rana pipiens,* 22°C (72°F)[308]
2.5 mg/kg IM q 72 hr	Mud puppy, waterdog, *Necturus* spp., 2–3°C (36–37°F)[309]

Itraconazole

23.5 mg/kg PO q 24 hr for three treatments maintains blood levels for another 5 days	Spiney lizards, *Sceloporus* sp., ambient temperature

Ketoconazole

15 mg/kg PO q 24 hr	Gopher tortoises, *Gopherus polyphemus,* 27°C (81°F)[310]

Metronidazole

20 mg/kg PO q 48 hr	Yellow rat snakes, *Elaphe obsoleta quadrivitatta*[311] Green iguanas, *Iguana iguana,* 31–34°C (88–93°F)[312] For anaerobic bacteria or protozoan overgrowth. Can give as whole tablets or crushed and suspended in water.[313] Discontinue if central nervous symptoms develop. For small patients injectable metronidazole (Metronidazole Redi-infusion, 5 mg/ml, Elkin-Sinn Inc.) works well.[314]

Piperacillin

80–100 mg/kg IM q 48 hr	Blood python, *Python curtus,* 28–30°C (82–86°F)[315]

continued

Empirically Derived Drug Dosages

Drug Dose/Route/Interval	Use/Comments/Reference
ENDOPARASITES	
Fenbendazole	
25–100 mg/kg PO q 14 days x four treatments	Drug of choice for nematodes[316]
Ivermectin	
0.2 mg/kg PO, SC q 14 days x four treatments	Can cause neurologic symptoms in some species, not recommended for skinks, DO NOT USE IN CHELONIANS.[286,317]
2.0 mg/kg cutaneuosly (anterior dorsal coelom)	Treatment for nematodes in frogs[316]
Praziquantel	
3–8 mg/kg PO, IM, repeat in 14 days	Drug of choice for trematodes[286,318]
Metronidazole	
100 mg/kg PO once	For appetite stimulation[16]
ECTOPARASITES	
Permectrin II	
0.007 to 0.002% spray q 14 days for three treatments	Treatment for mites. Dilute from 10% stock solution to 0.007% (5 ml in 710 ml tap water) to 0.002% (15 ml in 710 ml tap water) and use as spray, (Permectrin II, Bio-Centic Division, Boehringer Ingelheim Animal Health Inc.). Make fresh for each treatment.[319]
Ivermectin	
5 mg tap water solution	Spray for mites, do not use on chelonians. Mix new monthly.[320]

METABOLIC BONE DISEASE

Neo-calglucon (Calcium glubionate)

1 ml/kg PO q 12 hr for 1 to 3 months	Part of treatment for metabolic bone disease (MBD)[321,322]

10% Calcium gluconate

100 mg/kg (100 mg/ml) q 6 hr	For control of hypocalcemic muscle tremors, seizures, or flaccid paresis in lizards. As soon as patient is stable, switch to oral Neo-calglucon.

Calcitonin

50 IU/kg/wk IM for two treatments	Part of treatment for MBD. **Do not give if hypocalcemic** (plasma calcium < 8.5 mg/dl) or delay giving until 3 days of Neo-calglucon treatment.[322,323]

Vitamin D

1000 IU/kg IM for two treatments	Part of treatment for MBD.[320,321] Only indicated if history suggests vitamin D deficiency.

MISCELLANEOUS

Vitamin A

2000 IU/kg q 7–14 days SC, IM for two to four treatments	For treatment of hypovitaminosis A if clinical signs and dietary history support diagnosis. Overdosage will cause epidermal sloughing, dose carefully.[16,314]

Vitamin B complex

25 mg/kg PO q 24 hr for three to seven treatments	For treatment of thiamine deficiency and appetite stimulation, dosed on thiamine content.[16]

Oxytocin

2–10 IU/kg IM q 4–6 hr for one to three treatments	For egg retention, works well in chelonians. Provide warm, quiet, darkened environment with appropriate nesting substrate. Oviductal rupture has been reported with multiple doses.[324]

continued

Arginine vasotocin

0.01–1.0 micrograms/kg IV or intracoelomically	More efficacious than oxytocin in stimulating oviposition. Short shelf life unless frozen, expensive, experimental drug license and number required (Sigma Chemicals).[325]

Trimethoprim-sulfadiazine

30 mg/kg IM q 24 hr for two treatments, then q 48 hr	Good activity against gram-positive and -negative aerobes, especially in enteric infections. Not clear if bactericidal or bacteristatic in reptiles.[286]

ANESTHETICS

Lidocaine

1–2 % solution	Infiltrate to effect. Excellent for minor procedures.

Ketamine HCl

Painful at injection site, some reptiles may have an immediate or delayed violent reaction to injection. Should not be used with renal impairment. Larger reptiles require smaller mg/kg doses than smaller reptiles. Go to isoflurane for surgical anesthesia, analgesia is questionable, local anesthetic should be used in conjunction with ketamine.[326–328]

12–25 mg/kg IM	Crocodilians
30–50 mg/kg IM	Lizards, for light sedation then go to isoflurane for anesthesia
20–60 mg/kg IM	Snakes, light sedation
60–80 mg/kg IM	Snakes, light anesthesia
50–70 mg/kg IM	Turtles, sedation
70–100 mg/kg IM	Turtles, light anesthesia

Tiletamine HCl/Zolazepam HCl (Telazol)

Can be refrigerated for reuse up to 1 month after reconstitution. Severe respiratory depression possible, ventilate until spontaneously breathing. [300,320,328]

3–5 mg/kg IM	Crocodilians
5–10 mg/kg IM	Lizards, snakes
10–20 mg/kg IM	Turtles

Propofol, Disoprofol

Jugular vein and dorsal tail vein are easiest sites for administration in chelonians. White opaque liquid easily passed through small-gauge needle (27 gauge). Not painful with injection and perivascular injection does not cause problems. Induction is rapid (within 1 to 5 minutes) and smooth recovery is complete within 25 to 40 minutes. Surgical anesthesia lasts 15 to 25 minutes, making this an excellant anesthetic for short procedures or induction. However, intravenous administration may limit its usefulness. See Divers[265] and Bennett[330] for more information. Can be given intraosseously.[330]

12–15 mg/kg IV	All species

Isoflurane

Anesthetic of choice for surgery. Intubation and intermittent positive pressure ventilation advisable. Mask induction possible, or one can preanesthetize with low dose of ketamine, telazol, or propofol. Use 1–3% for maintenance, 3–5% for induction. If intubation desired, premedicate with atropine sulfate (0.04 mg/kg SC or IM) or glycopyrrolate (0.01 mg/kg SC or IM) 30 minutes prior to intubation. Nonrebreathing circuit advisable for reptiles < 10 kg with a minimum oxygen flow rate of 300 to 500 ml/kg/min, monitor EKG.

References

1. Boyer TH. A practitioner's guide to reptilian husbandry and care. Lakewood, CO: American Animal Hospital Association, 1993.

2. Mader DR, ed. Reptile medicine and surgery. Philadelphia: W.B. Saunders, 1996.

3. Ackerman LW. The biology, husbandry, and health care of reptiles. Neptune City, NJ: TFH Publications, 1997.

4. Barnard SM, Upton SJ. A veterinary guide to the parasites of reptiles, Vol. 1. Protozoa. Malabar, FL: Krieger, 1994.

5. Frye FL. Reptiles clinician's handbook. A compact clinical and surgical reference. Malabar, FL: Krieger, 1995.

6. Frye FL, Williams DL. Self-assessment color review of reptiles and amphibians. Ames, IA: Iowa State University Press, 1995.

7. McArthur S. Veterinary management of tortoises and turtles. Oxford: Blackwell Science, 1996.

8. Messonnier SW. Common reptile diseases and treatment. Cambridge, MA: Blackwell Science, 1996.

9. Rossi J, Rossi R. What's wrong with my snake? Lakeside, CA: Advanced Vivarium Systems, 1996.

10. Youngprapakorn P, Osavaaplangchai L, Kanchanapangka S. A color atlas of diseases of the crocodile. Thailand: Style Creative House, 1994.

11. Wright KM, Whittaker B. Amphibian medicine and captive husbandry. Malabar, FL: Krieger, 1998.

12. Frye FL. 1991. Biomedical and surgical aspects of captive reptile husbandry, 2nd ed, Vols. I and 2. Malabar, FL: Kreiger, 1991.

13. Frye FL. Biomedical and surgical aspects of captive reptile husbandry. Edwardsville, KS: VetMed Publishing, 1981.

14. Beynon PH, Lawton MPC, Cooper JE, eds. Manual of reptiles. Cheltenham, UK: British Small Animal Veterinary Association, 1992.

15. Cooper JE, Jackson OF, eds. Diseases of the reptilia, Vols. 1 and 2. London: Academic Press, 1981.

16. Frye FL. A practical guide for feeding captive reptiles. Malabar, FL: Kreiger, 1991.

17. Reichenbach-Klinke HH, Elkan E. The principal diseases of lower vertebrates. Book II: Diseases of amphibians. Book III: Diseases of reptiles. Neptune City: TFH Publications, 1965.

18. Marcus L. Veterinary biology and medicine of captive amphibians and reptiles. Philadelphia: Lea & Febebinger, 1981.

19. Hoff GL, Frye FL, Jacobson ER, eds. Diseases of amphibians and reptiles. New York: Plenum, 1984.

20. Ross RA, Marzec G. The bacterial disease of reptiles: their epidemiology, control, diagnosis and treatment. Stanford: Institute for Herpetological Research, 1984.

21. Murphy JB, Collins JT. A review of the diseases and treatments of captive turtles. Lawrence, KS: AMS, 1983.

22. Wallach JD, Boever WJ. Diseases of exotic animals. Philadelphia: W.B. Saunders, 1983.

23. Fowler ME, ed. Zoo and wild animal medicine, 2nd ed (1986), and Current therapy (1994). Philadelphia: W.B. Saunders.

24. Jacobson ER, Kollias G Jr. Exotic animals. New York: Churchill Livingstone, 1988.

25. Cooper JE, Hutchinson MF, Jackson OF, Maurice RJ, eds. 1985. Manual of exotic pets. Cheltenham, UK: British Small Animal Veterinary Association, 1985.

26. Fox JG, Cohen BJ, eds. Laboratory animal medicine. Orlando, FL: Academic Press, 1984.

27. Johnson-Delaney CA. Exotic animal medicine in practice, Vol. 1. Lake Worth, FL: Wingers, 1995.

28. Gillispie D. Reptiles. In Birchard SJ, Sherding RG, eds. Saunders manual of small animal practice. Philadelphia: W.B. Saunders, 1994.

29. Hawkey C, Bennett T. Atlas of comparative veterinary hematology. Ames, IA: Iowa State University Press, 1989.

30. Rubel GA, Isenbugel E, Wolvekamp P, eds. Atlas of diagnostic radiology of exotic pets. Philadelphia: W.B. Saunders, 1991.

31. Murphy JB, Collins JT, eds. Reproductive biology and diseases of captive reptiles. Oxford, OH: Society for the Study of Reptiles and Amphibians, 1980. Contributions to Herpetology No. 1.

32. Merck veterinary manual, 6th, 7th, 8th eds. Rahway, NJ: Merck and Co., 1986, 1993, 1998.

33. Kirk RE, ed. Current veterinary therapy, Vols. IV–XI. Philadelphia: W.B. Saunders.

34. Oldham JC, Smith HM. Laboratory anatomy of the iguana. Dubuque, IA: Wm. C Brown, 1975.

35. Ashley LM. Laboratory anatomy of the turtle. Dubuque, IA: Wm. C. Brown, 1962.

36. Chiasson RB. Laboratory anatomy of the alligator. Dubuque, IA: Wm. C. Brown, 1962.

37. Chiasson RB. Laboratory anatomy of *Necturus*. Dubuque, IA: Wm. C. Brown, 1969.

38. Underhill RA. Laboratory anatomy of the frog. Dubuque, IA: Wm. C. Brown, 1975.

39. Stuart RS. The anatomy of the bull frog, 4th ed. Chicago: Denoyer-Geppert, 1958 Co.

40. Bellairs A. The life of reptiles, Vols. 1 and 2. New York: Universe Books, 1970.

41. Gans C, et al, eds. The biology of the reptilia, Vols. 1–19. London: Academic Press, 1969–1997.

42. Halliday TR, Adler K. The encyclopedia of reptiles and amphibians. New York: Facts on File, 1986.

43. Cogger HG, Zweifel RC, eds. Reptiles & amphibians. New York: Smithmark, 1992.

44. Grzimek B, et al, eds. Grizmek's animal life encyclopedia: Vol. 5, Fishes II and amphibia, Vol. 6, Reptiles. New York: Van Nostrand Reinhold, 1972.

45. Beltz E, ed. Care in captivity: husbandry techniques for amphibians and reptiles. Chicago: Chicago Herpetological Society, 1989.

46. Mattison C. The care of reptiles and amphibians in captivity, 2nd ed rev. London: Blandford Press, 1987.

47. Townson S, Millichamp NJ, Lucas DGD, Millwood AJ, eds. The care and breeding of captive reptiles. London: British Herpetological Society, 1980.

48. Townson S, Lawrence K, eds. Reptiles. Breeding, behavior and veterinary aspects. London: British Herpetological Society, 1985.

49. Coote J, ed. Reptiles. Proceedings of the 1986 U.K. Herpetological Societies Symposium on Captive Breeding. London: British Herpetological Society, 1986.

50. Coote J, ed. Reptiles. Proceedings of the 1988 U.K. Herpetological Societies Symposium on Captive Breeding. London: British Herpetological Society, 1988.

51. Palazzolo C. 1996. Adding reptiles to your veterinary practice. In Mader DR, ed. Reptile medicine and surgery. Philadelphia: W.B. Saunders, 1996:1–8.

52. Barten SL. 1996. Reference sources for reptile clinicians. In Mader DR, ed. Reptile medicine and surgery. Philadelphia: W.B. Saunders, 1996:33–8.

53. Cooper JE, Lawton MPC. Introduction. In Beynon PH, Lawton MPC, Cooper JE, eds. Manual of reptiles. Cheltenham, UK: British Small Animal Veterinary Association, 1992.

54. Klauber LM. Rattlesnakes: Their habits, life histories and influence on mankind, Vols. 1 and 2. Berkeley, CA: University of California Press, 1972.

55. Boyer DM. Watering techniques for captive reptiles and amphibians. In Peterson KH, ed. 10th International Herpetological Symposium on Captive Propagation and Husbandry. Thurmont, MD: Zoological Consortium, 1986.

56. Barnett SL. 1997. Think up: meeting the needs of arboreal lizards. Proceedings of the Association of Reptilian and Amphibian Veterinarians, 1997:41–55.

57. Anonymous. Vitamin tolerance of animals. Subcommittee on Vitamin Tolerance, Committee on Animal Nutrition, Board of Agriculture, National Research Council. Washington, DC: National Academy Press, 1987:11–21.

58. Divers SJ. The captive husbandry and breeding of the green iguana (*Iguana iguana*): Parts 1 and 2. Rept Mag 1992;2(1–2):7–13, 24–32.

59. Packard GC, Phillip JA. The importance of the physical environment for the incubation of reptilian eggs. Contrib Herpetol 1994;11:195–208.

60. Tryon B. How to incubate reptile eggs: a proven technique. Herpetology 1975;3:33–7.

61. Hammack S. New concepts in colubrid egg incubation: a preliminary report. 15th International Symposium on Captive Propagation Husbandry, 1991.

62. Therac J. The incubation of the eggs of popular colubrids. Vivarium 1997;8(4):24–5, 56.

63. Angulo F. Here we go again? Reptile associated salmonellosis in humans. Fourth Annual Proceedings of the Association of Reptilian and Amphibian Veterinarians, 1997:65–6.

64. Grier JW, Bjerke MS, Nolan LK. Snakes and the *Salmonella* situation. Bull Chicago Herp Soc 1993;28(3):53–9.

65. Morse EV, Duncan MA. Salmonellosis—an environmental health problem. J Am Vet Med Assoc 1974;165:1015–19.

66. Evans R. Follow-up on salmonellosis in exotic pets. Prof Anim Lab News 1995;3(4):8–12.

67. Chiodini RJ, Sundberg JP. Salmonellosis in reptiles: a review. Am J Epidemiol 1981;113:494–9.

68. Johnson-Delaney CA. Reptile zoonoses and threats to public health. In Mader DR, ed. Reptile medicine and surgery. Philadelphia: W.B. Saunders, 1996:20–33.

69. Centers for Disease Control and Prevention. Reptile-associated salmonellosis— selected states. MMWR Morbid Mortal Wkly Rep 1994–1995;44):347–50.

70. Jacobson ER. Veterinary procedures for acquisition and release of captive-bred hepetofauna. Contrib Herpetol 1994;11:109–18.

71. Jacobson ER. An update on inclusion body disease of boid snakes. Fourth Annual Proceedings of the Association of Reptilian and Amphibian Veterinarians, 1997:165.

72. Boycott RC, Bourquin O. The South African tortoise book. Johannesburg: Southern Book Publishers, 1988.

73. Highfield AC. Practical encyclopedia of keeping and breeding tortoises and freshwater turtles. London: Carapace Press, 1996.

74. Jarchow JL. Hibernating your turtle safely. Notes North Ohio Assoc Herpetol 1993;20(11):8–11.

75. de Vosjoli P. The general care and maintenance of box turtles. Lakeside, CA: Advanced Vivarium Systems, 1991.

76. Boyer TH, Boyer DM. Biology: Turtles, tortoises and terrapins. In Mader DR, ed. Reptile medicine and surgery. Philadelphia: W.B. Saunders, 1996:69–78.

77. NYTS. 1990. Guidelines for the housing of turtles and tortoises: minimum standard housing guidelines for pet shops, wholesale animal dealers, and other commercial establishments. New York: New York Turtle and Tortoise Society, 1990:19:insert.

78. Boyce WA, Cardeilhac P, Lane T, Buergelt C, King M. Sebekiosis in captive alligator hatchlings. J Am Vet Med Assoc 1984;185:1419–20.

79. Jackson OF. Weight and measurement data on tortoises (*Testudo graeca* and *Testudo hermanni*) and their relationship to health. J Small Anim Pract 1980;21:409.

80. Donoghue S, Langenburg J. Nutrition. In Mader DR, ed. Reptile medicine and surgery. Philadelphia: W.B. Saunders, 1996:149–74.

81. Jackson OF, Lawrence K. Chelonians. In Manual of exotic pets, rev ed. Cheltenham, UK: British Small Animal Veterinary Association, 1985.

82. Jacobson ER, Weinstein M, Berry K, Hardenbrook B, Tomlinson C, Frietas D. Problems with using weight versus carapace length relationships to assess tortoise health. Vet Rec 1993;132:222–3.

83. Donoghue S. Nutritional status of tortoises: using morphometrics to assess body condition. Vivarium 1997;8(2):46–9.

84. Lawrence K, Hawkey C. Seasonal variation in hematological data from Mediterranean tortoises, *Testudo graeca* and *Testudo hermanni*, in captivity. Res Vet Sci 1986;40;225–30.

85. Gottdenker NL, Jacobson ER. Effect of venipuncture sites on hematologic and clinical biochemical values in desert tortoises (*Gopherus agassizii*). Am J Vet Res 1995;56:1921.

86. Crawshaw GJ, Holz P. Comparison of plasma biochemical values in blood and blood-lymph mixtures from red-eared sliders, *Trachemys scripta elegans.* Bull Assoc Rept Amphib Vet 1996;6(2):7–9.

87. Owens DM, Ruiz GJ. New methods of obtaining blood and cerebral spinal fluid from marine turtles. Herpetologia 1980;36(1):17–20.

88. Jacobson ER, Schumacher J, Green M. Field and clinical techniques for sampling and handling blood for hematologic and selected biochemical determinations in the desert tortoise, *Xerobates agassizii.* Copeia 1992;(1):237–41.

89. Jarchow JL. Hospital care of the reptile patient. In Jacobson E, Kollias G Jr, eds. Exotic animals. New York: Churchill Livingstone, 1988:19–34.

90. Prezant RM, Jarchow JL. Lactated fluid use in reptiles: Is there a better solution? Proceedings of the ARAV Annual Conference, Houston, 1997:83–7.

91. Murray MJ. Pneumonia and normal respiratory function. In Mader DR, ed. Reptile medicine and surgery. Philadelphia: W.B. Saunders, 1996:396–405.

92. Boyer TH. Common problems of box turtles (*Terrapene* spp) in captivity. Bull Assoc Rept Amphib Vet 1992;2(1):9.

93. Elkan E, Zwart P. The ocular disease of young terrapins caused by vitamin A deficiency. Pathol Vet 1967;4:201.

94. Boyer TH. Differential diagnosis by symptoms: turtles, tortoises and terrapins. In Mader DR, ed. Reptile medicine and surgery. Philadelphia: W.B. Saunders, 1996:332–6.

95. Boyer TH. Hypovitaminosis A and hypervitaminosis A. In Mader DR, ed. Reptile medicine and surgery. Philadelphia: W.B. Saunders, 1996:382–3.

96. Jacobson ER, Gaskin JM, Brown MB, Harris RK, Gardiner CH, LaPointe JL, Adams HP, Reggiardo C. Chronic upper respiratory tract disease of free-ranging desert tortoises (*Xerobates agassizii*). J Wildl Dis 1991;27:296–316.

97. Lawerence K, Needham JR. Rhinitis in long term captive Mediterranean tortoises (*Testudo graeco* and *Testudo hermanni*). Vet Rec 1985;117:662–4.

98. Jacobson ER. The desert tortoise and upper respiratory tract disease. Bull Assoc Rept Amphib Vet 1994;4(1):6–7.

99. Jacobson ER, et al. Herpes-like infection in Argentine tortoises. J Am Vet Med Asssoc 1985;187:1227.

100. Muller M, Sachsse W, Zangger. Herpesvirus-epidemie bei der griechischen (*Testudo hermanni*) und der maurischen Landschildkrote (*T. graeca*) in der Schweiz. Schweiz Arch Tierheilkd 1990;132:199.

101. Pettman KCB, Drew ME, Ramsey E, et al. Herpesvirus-like particles associated with respiratory disease in a California desert tortoises (*Xerobates agassizii*). Proc Am Assoc Zoo Vets 1991;157.

102. Jacobson ER. Diseases of reptiles: parts I and II. Comp Cont Ed 1981;122:124–97.

103. Bennett RA. Reptilian surgery, parts I and II. Comp Cont Ed 1989;11:10–20, 122–34.

104. Harwell G. Repair of injuries to the chelonian plastron and carapace. In Kirk RW, ed. Current veterinary therapy X. Philadelphia: W.B. Saunders, 1989:789.

105. Isaza R, Jacobson ER. Non-nutritional bone diseases in reptiles. In Current veterinary therapy XII. Philadelphia: W.B. Saunders, 1995:1357–61.

106. Gould WJ, Georgi ME. Myiasis in two box turtles. J Am Vet Med Assoc 1991;199:1067.

107. Mader DR. Chelonian medicine. Proceedings of the Midwest Veterinary Conference 1993:262.

108. Silverman S, Janssen DL. In Mader DR, ed. Reptile medicine and surgery. Philadelphia: W.B. Saunders, 1996:258–64.

109. Barten SL. Paraphimosis. In Mader DR, ed. Reptile medicine and surgery. Philadelphia: W.B. Saunders, 1996:395–6.

110. Mautino M, Page CD. Biology and medicine of turtles and tortoises. Vet Clin North Am 1993;23:1251.

111. McArthur S. Veterinary management of tortoises and turtles. Oxford: Blackwell Science, 1996.

112. Barten SL. Personal communication, 1992–1993. Vernon Hills Animal Hospital, 1260 Butterfield Road, Mundelein, IL 60060.

113. Bennett RA, Mader DR. Soft tissue surgery. In Mader DR, ed. Reptile medicine and surgery. Philadelphia: W.B. Saunders, 1996:287–98.

114. Keymer IF. Diseases of chelonians: necropsy survey of tortoises. Vet Rec 1978;103:548.

115. Highfield AC. Keeping and breeding tortoises in captivity. Avon, England: R & A Pub., 1990.

116. Cooper J, Beynon PH , eds. Manual of exotic pets, 3rd ed. Cheltenham, UK: British Small Animal Veterinary Association, 1991.

117. Lawton MPC. In Beynon PH, Lawton MP., Cooper JE, eds. manual of reptiles. Cheltenham, UK: British Small Animal Veterinary Association, 1992.

118. Divers S J. Captive husbandry of Mediterranean tortoises (*Testudo graeco* and *Testudo hermanni*). Proceedings of the Association of Reptilian and Amphibian Veterinarians, 1996:31–35.

119. Tear JA, Bush M. Toxicity and efficacy of ivermectin in chelonians. J Am Vet Med Assoc 1983;183:1195–7.

120. Jacobson ER. Reptiles. Vet Clin North Am 1987;17-1203–25.

121. Rideout BA, Montali RJ, Phillips LG, Gardiner GH. Mortality of captive tortoises due to viviparous nematodes of the genus *Proatractis* (family Atractidae). J Wildl Dis 23(1):103–8.

122. Conboy GA, Laursen JR, Averbeck GA, Stromberg be. Diagnostic guide to some helminth parasites of aquatic turtles. Comp Cont Ed 1993;15:1217–21.

123. Jacobson, ER, Clubb S, Greiner E. Amebiasis in red-footed tortoises. J Am Vet Med Assoc 1983; 183(11):1192–1194.

124. Wright K. Common medical problems of tortoises. Proc North Am Vet Conf 1997;11:769–71.

125. Frye FL. Personal Communication, 1994. FL Frye and Associates, Veterinary Medical Surgical and Pathology Consultation, 741 Plum Lane, Davis, CA 95616.

126. de Vosjoli P. The general care and maintenance of red-eared sliders and other popular freshwater turtles. Lakeside, CA: Advanced Vivarium Systems, 1992.

127. de Vosjoli P. The general care and maintenance of poular tortoises. Santee, CA: Advanced Vivarium Systems, 1996.

128. Ernst CH, Barbour RW. Turtles of the world. Washington: Smithsonian Institution Press, 1989:. 194-7.

129. Pritchard P. Encyclopedia of turtles. Neptune City, NJ: TFH Publications, 1979.

130. Swingland IR, Klemens MW, eds. The conservation and biology of tortoises. Gland, Switzerland: International Union for the Conservation of Nature and Natural Resources, 1989.

131. Rodda GH. The mating behavior of *Iguana iguana*. Washington, DC: Smithsonian Institution Press, 1992. Smithsonian Contributions in Zoology No. 534.

132. Rand AS, et al. The diet of a generalized folivore: *Iguana iguana* in Panama. J Herpetol 1990;24:211–4.

133. Troyer, K. Diet selection and digestion in *Iguana iguana*: the importance of age and nutrient requirements. Oecologica 1984;61:201–7.

134. Hirth HE. Some aspects of the natural history *Iguana iguana* on a tropical strand. Ecology 1963;44:613–5.

135. Loftin H, Tyson E. Iguanas as carrion eaters. Copeia 1965;4:515.

136. Fitzgerald K. Personal communication, 1996. Alameda East Veterinary Hospital, Aurora, CO.

137. de Vosjol P. The green iguana manual. Lakeside: Advanced Vivarium Systems, 1992.

138. Miller T. Artificial incubation of eggs of the green iguana (*Iguana iguana*). Zoo Biol 1987;6:225–36.

139. Bock BC, Rand AS, Burghardt GM. Nesting season movements of female green iguanas (*Iguana iguana*) in Panama. Copeia 1989;1:214–6.

140. Werner DI, Miller TJ. Artificial nests for female green iguanas. Herp Rev 1984;15:57–8.

141. Frye FL, Townsend W. Iguanas: a guide to their biology and captive care. Malabar, FL: Krieger, 1993.

142. Frye FL. Personal communication, 1992. FL Frye and Associates, Veterinary Medical Surgical and Pathology Consultation, 741 Plum Lane, Davis, CA 95616.

143. Beltz E, ed. Care in captivity: husbandry techniques for amphibians and reptiles. Chicago: Chicago Herpetological Society, 1989.

144. Anderson NL. Husbandry and clinical evaluation of *Iguana iguana*. Comp Cont Ed 1991;113:1265.

145. de Vosjoli P. General care and maintenance of the green iguana. Lakeside, CA: Advanced Vivarium Systems, 1990:1–32.

146. Barten SL. Diseases of the green iguana, *Iguana iguana*. North American Vet Conference Proceedings, 1996:811–19.

147. Boyer TH. Green iguana care. Bull Assoc Amphib Rept Vet 1992;1:124.

148. Barten SL. Lizards. In Mader DR, ed. Reptile medicine and surgery. Philadelphia: W.B. Saunders, 1996:47–61.

149. Donoghue S. Fact vs. Fiction: clarifying and verifying the literature and conversations on the Internet. Proceedings 2nd Annual ARAV Conference, Sacramento, 1995.

150. Jacobson ER. In Beynon PH, Lawton MPC, Cooper JE, eds.1992. Manual of reptiles. Cheltenham, UK: British Small Animal Veterinary Association, 1992.

151. Lawton MPC. Hands free, non-chemical restraint of Iguanidae for radiography. Fourth Annual Proceedings Association of Reptilian Amphibian Veterinarians, 1997:1–3.

152. Jarchow JL. Hospital care of the reptile patient. In Jacobson JE, Kollias GV, eds. Exotic animals. New York: Churchill Livingstone, 1988:19–34.

153. Bennett RA. Intraosseous catheters in small mammals, Orlando, FL: Proceedings NA Vet Conf, 1996; 10:847.

154. Donoghue S, Langenberg J. Nutrition. In Mader DR, ed. Reptile medicine and surgery. Philadelphia: W.B. Saunders, 1996:148–73.

155. Boyer TH. Metabolic bone disease. In Mader DR, ed. Reptile medicine and surgery. Philadelphia: WB Saunders, 1996:385–92.

156. Mader DR. Metabolic bone disease in captive reptiles. Vivarium 1990;2:12–13.

157. Barten SL. The medical care of iguanas and other common pet lizards. Vet Clin North Am 1993;23:1213–49.

158. Mader DR. Use of calcitonin in green iguanas, *Iguana iguana*, with metabolic bone disease. Bull Assoc Rept Amphib Vet 1993;3(1):5.

159. Bennett RA. Fracture management. In Mader DR, ed. Reptile medicine and surgery. Philadelphia : W.B. Saunders, 1996:281–7.

160. Boyer TH, Getzy D, Vap L, Innis C. Clinicopathologic findings of twelve cases of renal failure in *Iguana iguana*. Proceedings of the Association of Reptilian and Amphibian Veterinarians, 1996;113.

161. Jarchow JL. Personal communication, 1997. Sonora Animal Hospital, Tucson, AZ 85705.

162. Massry SG. Divalent ion metabolism and renal osteodystrophy. In Massry SG, Glassock RJ, eds. Textbook of nephrology, 3rd ed, Vol. 2. Baltimore, MD:Williams & Wilkins, 1995:1467–9.

163. Salusky IB, Ramirez JA, Coburn JW. The renal osteodystrophies. In DeGroot LJ, ed. Endocrinology, 3rd ed. Philadelphia, PA: W.B. Saunders, 1995:1162–3.

164. Rossi JV. Gastrointestinal problems of the green iguana. Proceedings of the North American Veterinary Conference, Orlando, FL, 1997:756.

165. Mader DR. Reproductive surgery in the green iguana. Semin Avian Exotic Pet Med 1996;5(4):214–21.

166. Maxwell LK, Greiner EG. Nematode parasites of iguanine lizards. Proceedings of the Association of Reptilian and Amphiban Veterinarians, 1997:57–9.

167. Frye FL, Mader DR, Centofanti BV. Interspecific (lizard:human) sexual aggression in captive iguanas (*Iguana iguana*): a preliminary compilation of eighteen cases. Bull Assoc Amphib Rept Vet 1991;1(1):46.

168. Hatfield JW. Green iguana, the ultimate owner's manual. Portland: Dunthorpe Press, 1996.

169. Frye FL. *Iguana iguana,* guide for sucessful captive care. Malabar, FL: Krieger, 1995.

170. Webb GJ, Hollis GJ, Manolis SC. Feeding, growth, and food conversion rates of wild juvenile saltwater crocodiles (*Crocodylus porosus*) J Herpetol 1991;25:462–3.

171. Avery HW, et al. Roles of diet protein and temperature in the growth and nutritional energetics of juvenile slider turtles, *Trachemys scripta.* Pysiol Zool 1993; 66:902–25.

172. Barker D. Preliminary observations on nutrient composition differences between adult and pinhead crickets, *Acheta domestica.* Bull Assoc Rept Amphib Vet 1997;7(1):10–3.

173. Allen ME, Oftedal OT. Dietary manipulation of the calcium content of feed crickets. J Zoo Anim Med 1989;26–33.

174. Strzelwicz M, et al. Feeding insectivores: increasing the calcium content of wax moth larvae. J Zoo Anim Med 1985;16:25–7.

175. Zwart P, Rulkens RJ. Improving the calcium content of mealworms. Int Zoo Yrbk 1979;19:254–5.

176. Frye FL, Calvert C. Preliminary information on the nutritional content of mulberry silk moth (*Bombyx mori*) larvae. J Zoo Wildl Med 1989;20:73–5.

177. Frye FL. Captive invertebrates: a guide to their biology and husbandry. Malabar, FL: Krieger, 1992.

178. Dierenfeld ES, Barker E. Nutrient composition of whole prey commonly fed to reptiles and amphibians. Proceedings of the Association of Reptilian and Amphibian Veterinarians, 1995:3–15.

179. Donoghue S. Clinical nutrition of reptiles and amphibians. Proceedings of the Association of Reptilian and Amphibian Veterinarians, 1995:16–37.

180. Allen ME, Oftedal OT. The nutrition of carnivorous reptiles. Contrib Herpetol 1994;11:71–82.

181. Rossi JV, Rossi R. Snakes of the United States and Canada, Vol. 2, Western area. Malabar, FL: Krieger, 1995.

182. Veer V, Ciszar D, Smith H. Preference for formerly frozen mice over freshly euthanized mice by captive snakes of seven species from famalies Boidae and Colubridae. Vivarium 1996;7(6):18.

183. Rossi JV. Snakes of the United States and Canada, Vol. 1, Eastern area. Malabar, FL: Krieger, 1992.

184. de Vosjoli P. The general care and maintenance of Burmese pythons. Lakeside, CA: Advanced Vivarium Systems, 1991.

185. de Vosjoli P. In support of the keeping of boas and pythons by the private sector. Vivarium 1992;4(4):34–45.

186. Applegate R. The general care and maintenence of milk snakes. Lakeside, CA: Advanced Vivarium Systems, 1992.

187. Barker DG, Barker TM. Pythons of the world, Vol. 1, Australia. Lakeside, CA: Advanced Vivarium Systems, 1994.

188. de Vosjoli P. The general care and maintenance of ball pythons, Lakeside, CA: Advanced Vivarium Systems, 1990.

189. de Vosjoli P, Barker D, Klingenberg R, Barker T. The ball python manual. Lakeside, CA: Advanced Vivarium Systems, 1994.

190. Greene HW. Snakes: The evolution of mystery in nature. Berkeley: University of California Press, 1997.

191. Kauffeld C. Snakes: The keeper and the kept. Garden City, NY: Doubleday, 1969.

192. McEchern MJ. Keeping and breeding corn snakes. Lakeside, CA: Advanced Vivarium Systems, 1991.

193. Mehrtens J. Living snakes of the world. New York: Sterling, 1987.

194. Perlowin D. The general care and maintenance of garter snakes and water snakes. Lakeside, CA: Advanced Vivarium Systems, 1994.

195. Ross RA, Marzec G. The reproductive husbandry of pythons and boas. Stanford, CA: Institute for Herpetological Research, 1990.

196. Shine R. Australian snakes, a natural history. Ithaca, NY: Cornell University Press, 1991.

197. Barten SL. Reptile physical examination. Proceedings of the North American Veterinary Conference. Gainesville: Eastern States Veterinary Association, 1996:809–10.

198. McCracken H. Reptilian hematology and blood chemistry. In Proceedings. Clinical Pathology, JD Stewart Memorial Refresher Course for Veterinarians, 1993:277–313.

199. Jacobson ER. Laboratory investigations. In Beynon PH, Lawton MPC, Cooper JE, eds. Manual of reptiles. Gloucestershire, UK: British Small Animal Veterinary Association, 1992:50–4.

200. Olson GA, Hessler JR, Faith RE. Techniques for blood collection and intravascular infusion of reptiles. Lab Anim Sci 1975;25:783–6.

201. Rosskopf WJ, Woerpel RW, Fudge A, Pitts BJ, Whittaker D. 1A practical method of performing venipuncture in snakes. VM/SAC, May: 1982:820–1.

202. Funk RS. 1996. Anorexia, vomiting and regurgitation. In Mader DR, ed. Reptile medicine and surgery. Philadelphia: W.B. Saunders, 1996:346–8, 425–6.

203. Klingenberg RJ. A comparison of fenbendazole and ivermectin for the treatment of nematode parasites in ball pythons, *Python regius*. Bull Assoc Rept Amphib Vet 1992;2:5–6.

204. Klingenberg RJ. Management of the anorectic ball python. Proceedings of the North American Veterinary Conference. Gainesville: Eastern States Veterinary Association, 1996:830.

205. Moyle M, Ross R. Problems encountered with the husbandry of the emerald tree boa, *Corallus canina*. Proceedings 15th International Herp. Symposium on Captive Prop. Husbandry, 1991:119–26.

206. Murray MJ. Pneumnia and normal respiratory function. In Mader DR, ed. Reptile medicine and surgery, Philadelphia: W.B. Saunders, 1996:396–405.

207. Boyer DM. Snake mite (*Ophionyssus natricus*) eradication utilizing permectrin spray. Bull Assoc Rept Amphib Vet 1995;5(1):4–5.

208. Mader DR. In Mader DR, ed. Reptile medicine and surgery. Philadelphia: W.B. Saunders, 1996.

209. Stahl SJ. Treatment and management of mites in snakes and lizards. Proceedings of the North American Veterinary Conference, 1997;11:757–8.

210. Stahl SJ. Inclusion body diease in boids. Rept Amphib Mag 1996;May/June:112–17.

211. Axthelm MK. Clinicopatholgic and virlogic observations of a probable viral disease affecting boid snakes. Proceedings of the American Association of Zoo Veterinarians, 1985;108.

212. Schumacher J, Jacobson ER, Homer BL, Gaskin JM. Inclusion body disease in boid snakes. J Zoo Wildl Med 1994;25(4):511–24.

213. Mader DR. Inclusion body diseases virus. Reptiles 1996;4(11):8–9.

214. Jacobson ER. An update on inclusion body disease of boid snakes. Proceedings of the Association of Reptilian and Amphibian Veterinarians, 1997:165.

215. Klingenberg R. IBD: Coming to your collection next? Vivarium 1997;8(4):38-41.

216. Clark HF, Lief FS, Lunger PD, et al. Fer-de-lance virus: a probable paramyxovirus isolated from a reptile. J Gen Virol 1979;44:405–18.

217. Jacobson ER. Update on ophidian paramyxovirus infections. AAZV/WDA/AAWV 1995:223.

218. Jacobson ER, Gaskin JM, Page D, Iverson WO, Johnson JW. Illness associated with paramyxo-like virus infection in a zoological collection of snakes. J Am Vet Med Assoc 1981;179:1227–30.

219. Jacobson ER, Gaskin JM, Flanagan JP, Odum RA. Antibody responses of western diamondback rattlesnakes (*Crotalus atrox*) to inactivated ophidian paramyxovirus vaccines. J Zoo Wildl Med 1991;22(2):184–90.

220. Lloyd ML, Flanagan J. Recent developments in ophidian paramyxovirus research and recommendations on control. Proc AAZV 1991:151–56.

221. Jacobson E, Gaskin JM, Simpson CF, Terrell TG. Paramyxo-like virus infection in a rock rattlesnake. J Am Vet Med Assoc 1980;177:796–9.

222. Flannagan J. Paramyxovirus infection of snakes. A report of the AAZV Infectious Disease Committee. AAZV, 1992:1–6.

223. Cranfield MR, Graczyk TK. Cryptosporidiosis. In Mader DR, ed. Reptile medicine and surgery. Philadelphia: W.B. Saunders, 1996:392–4.

224. Tilley M, Upton SJ, Freed PS. A comparative study on the biology of *Cryptosporidium serpentis* and *Cryptosporidium parvum* (Apicomplexa: Cryptosporidiidae). J Zoo Wildl Med 1990;21:463–7.

225. Brownstein DG, Sirandberg JD, Montail RJ, Bush M, Foriner J. *Cryptosporidium* in snakes with hypertrophic gastritis. Vet Pathol 1977;14:606–17.

226. Gillespie D. Cryptosporidiosis in reptiles. In Kirk RW, ed. Current vet therapy, Philadelphia: W.B. Saunders, 1986: 748-49.

227. Agnew DW. Cryptosporidiosis in reptiles—a review. AAV Infectious Disease Committee, AAZV, 1992:1–9.

228. Cook RA, Stetter M. Clinical challenge. J Zoo Anim Med 1988;19(1–2):60–1.

229. Godshalk CP, MacCoy DM, Patterson JS, McKiernan BC. Gastric hypertrophy associated with cryptosporidiosis in a snake. J Am Vet Med Assoc 1986;189:1126–8.

230. Cranfield MR, Graczyk. An update on ophidian cryptosporidiosis. Joint Conference AAZV/WDA/AAWV, 1995:225–30.

231. Carmel BP, Groves V. Chronic cryptosporidiosis in Australian elapid snakes: control of an outbreak in a captive colony. Aust Vet J 1993;70(8):293–5.

232. Barten SL. Oviductal rupture in a Burmese python (*Python molorus bivittatus*) treated with oxytocin for egg retention. J Zoo Anim Med 1985;16:141–3.

233. Klingenberg RJ. Egg-binding in colubrid snakes. Vivarium 1991;3:32–5.

234. Millichamp NJ, et al. Egg retention in snakes. J Am Vet Med Assoc 1983;183:1213–8.

235. Brown C, Martin R. Dystocia in snakes. Comp Cont Ed 1990;12:361–7.

236. Bolton M. The management of crocodiles in captivity. Rome: Food and Agriculture Organization of the United Nations, 1989.

237. Buenviaje GN, Ladds PW, Melville L, Manolis SC. Disease-husbandry associations in farmed crocodiles in Queensland and the Northern Territory. Aust Vet J 1994;71(6):165–73.

238. Thorbjarnarson JB. Diet of the spectacled caiman (*Caiman crocodilus*) in the central Venezuelan llanos. Herpetologica 1993;49(1):108–17.

239. Grahame JW, Webb W, Hollis GJ, Manolis SC. Feeding, growth and food conversion rates of wild juvenile saltwater crocodiles (*Crocodylus porosus*). J Herpetol 1991;25:462–73.

240. Jacobson ER. Immobilization, blood sampling, necropsy techniques and diseases of crocodilians: a review. J Zoo Anim Med 1984;15:38–45.

241. Wallach JD, Hoessle C. Steatitis in captive crocodilians. J Am Vet Med Assoc 1968;153:845–7.

242. Larsen RE, Buergelt C, Cardeilhac PT, Jacobson ER. Steatitis and fat necrosis in captive alligators. J Am Vet Med Assoc 1983;183:1202–4.

243. Oftedal OT, Boness DJ. Considerations in the use of fish as food. Annual Meeting of the American Association of Zoo Veterinarians, 1983:149–60.

244. Cardeilhac P. Nutritional disorders of alligators. Gainesville: First Annual Alligator Production Conference, 1981.

245. Jubb T. A thiamine responsive nervous disease in saltwater crocodiles (*Crocodylus porosus*). Vet Rec 1992;131:347–48.

246. Wallach JD, Hoessle C, Bennett J. Hypoglycemic shock in captive alligators. J Am Vet Med Assoc 1967;151:893–6.

247. Ladds PW, Mangunwirjo H, Sebayang D, Daniels PW. Diseases in young farmed crocodiles in Irian Jaya. Vet Rec 1995;136:121–4.

248. Boyce W, Cardeilhac P, Lane T, Buergelt C, Kinge M. Sebekiosis in captive alligator hatchlings. J Am Vet Med Assoc 1984;185:1419–20.

249. Horner RF. Poxvirus in farmed Nile crocodiles. Vet Rec 1988;122:459–62.

250. Pandey GS, Inque N, Ohshima K, Okada K. Poxvirus infection in Nile crocodiles (*Crocodylus niloticus*). Res Vet Sci 1990;49:171–6.

251. Glassman AB, Bennett CE, Hazen TC. Peripheral blood components in *Alligator mississippiensis*. Trans Am Microsc Soc 1981;100(2):210–15.

252. Ross CA, ed. Crocodiles and alligators. New York: Facts on File, 1989.

253. Webb GJW, Manolis SC, Whitehead PJ, eds. Wildlife management: crocodiles and alligators. NSW, Australia: Surrey Beatty & Sons, 1987.

254. Bonath K. Halothane inhalation anesthesia in reptiles and its clinical control. In Olney PJS, ed. International Zoo Yearbook, Vol. 19. London: Zoological Society of London, 1979:112–25.

255. Jackson OF, Cooper JE. Anesthesia and surgery. In Cooper JE, Jackson OF, eds. Diseases of the Reptilian, Vol. 2. London: Academic Press, 1981:535–9.

256. Rosenburg ME. Temperature and nervous conduction in the tortoise. J Physiol (Lond) 1978;289:83.

257. Holz P, et al. The reptilian renal portal system and its effects on drug kinetics. Pittsburgh: Proc Am Assoc Zoo Vets 1994:95–6.

258. Jacobson E. Reptiles. In Exotic pet medicine. Veterinary clinics of North America. Philadelphia: W.B. Saunders, 1987:1203–25.

259. Sedgwick C. Anesthetic and chemical restraint techniques for zoo animals and wildlife. Proceedings of the American Animal Hospital Association Annual Meeting, 1988:162–6.

260. Burke T. Reptile anesthesia. In Zoo and wild animal medicine. Philadelphia: W.B. Saunders, 1986:153–5.

261. Cooper JE. Ketamine hydrochloride as an anesthetic for East African reptiles. Vet Rec 1974;95:37–41.

262. Bennett RA. A review of anesthesia and chemical restraint in reptiles. J Zoo Wildl Med 1991;22(3):282–303.

263. Lawton MPC. Anesthesia. In Beynon PH, Lawton MPC, Cooper JE, eds. Manual of reptiles. Gloucestershire: BSAVA, 1992:170–83.

264. Divers SJ. The use of propofol in reptile anesthesia. Tampa: Proceedings of the Association of Reptilian and Amphibian Veterinarians, 1996:57–9.

265. Mader DR. Intravenous catheters. Orlando, FL: Proceedings of the North American Veterinary Conference, 1992:699–700.

266. Millichamp N. Surgical techniques in reptiles. In Jacobson E, Kollias G Jr, eds. Exotic animals. New York: Churchill Livingstone, 1988:49–59.

267. Bennett RA. Current techniques in reptile anesthesia. Proceedings of the North American Veterinary Conference, 1993:767–8.

268. Mader DR. Pulse oximetry as a tool for monitoring reptilian patients. Proceedings of the Association of Reptilian and Amphibian Veterinarians, 1995:81–2.

269. Bennett, RA. Anesthesia. In Mader DR, ed. Reptile medicine and surgery. Philadelphia: W.B. Saunders, 1996.

270. Schumacher J. Reptiles and amphibians. In Thurman JC, Tranquilli WJ, Benson GJ, eds. Lumb and Jones' veterinary anesthesia, 3rd ed. Baltimore: Williams & Wilkins, 1996:670–85.

271. Lawrence K. The use of antibiotics in reptiles: a review. J Small Anim Pract 1983;24:741–52.

272. Stewart JS. Anaerobic bacterial infections in reptiles. J Zoo Wildl Med 1990;21:180–4.

273. Holz P, et al. The reptilian renal portal system and its effects on drug kinetics. Pittsburgh: Proceedings of the American Association of Zoo Veterinarians, 1994:95–6.

274. Mader DR. Personal communication, 1994 and 1996. Long Beach Animal Hospital, Long Beach, CA.

275. Lawrence K. Drug dosages for chelonians. Vet Rec 1984;115.

276. Bush M, Smeller JM, Charache P, Soloron HM. Preliminary study of antibiotics in snakes. Proceedings of the American Association of Zoo Veterinarians, 1976.

277. Hodge MK. The effect of acclimation temperature on gentamicin nephrotoxicity in the Florida banded water snake (*Natrix fasciata*). American Association of Zoo Veterinarians Annual Proceedings, Knoxville, 1978: 78:226–37.

278. Mader DR, Conzelman GM, Baggot JD. Effects of ambient temperature on the half-life and dosage regimen of amikacin in the gopher snake. J Am Vet Med Assoc 1985;187:1134–6.

279. Caligiuri R, et al. The effects of ambient temperature on amikacin pharmacokinetics in gopher tortoises. J Vet Pharmacol Ther 1990;13:287–91.

280. Jacobson ER. Use of antimicrobials in reptiles. Proceedings Arizona, California, Nevada Veterinary Conference, 1994.

281. Lawrence K. The use of drugs in reptiles. Veterinary Manual, 26th ed. Grunsell G, Hill FWG, Raw M, eds. Bristol: John Wright & Sons, 1986.

282. Beehler BA, Sauro AM. Aerobic bacterial isolates and antibiotic sensitivities in a captive reptile population. Proceedings of the Association of Zoo Veterinarians, 1983:198–200.

283. Jacobson ER. Gentamicin-related visceral gout in two boid snakes. VetMed/Small Animal Clinic 1976;March:361–3.

284. Montali RJ, Bush M, Smeller JM. The pathology of neprotoxicity of gentamicin in snakes. Vet Pathol 1979;16:108–15.

285. Johnson JH, Jensen JM, Brumbaugh GW, Boothe DW. Amikacin pharmacokinetics and the effects of ambient temperature on the dosage regimen in ball pythons (*Python regius*). J Zoo Wildl Med 1997;28(1):80–8.

286. Jacobson ER. Use of chemotherapeutics in reptile medicine. In Jacobson E, Kollias G Jr, eds. Exotic animals. New York: Churchill Livingstone, 1988:35–48.

287. Mader DR. Antibiotic therapy in reptile medicine. In Frye FL. Biomedical and surgical aspects of captive reptile husbandry, 2nd ed, Vol. 2. Malabar, FL: Kreiger, 1991.

288. Klingenberg RJ. In Mader DR, ed. Reptile mdicine and surgery. Philadelphia: W.B. Saunders, 1996:299–321.

289. Bush M, Smeller JM, Charach P, Arthur R. Biological half-life of gentamicin in gopher snakes. Am J Vet Res 1978;39(1):171–3.

290. Teare JA, Bush M. Toxicity and efficacy of ivermectin in chelonians. J Am Vet Med Assoc 1983;183:1195–7.

291. Clark CH, Rogers ED, Milton JL. Plasma concentrations of chloramphenicol in snakes. Am J Vet Res 1985;46:2654–7.

292. Jacobson ER. Use of antimicrobial therapy in reptiles. In Antimicrobial therapy in caged birds and exotics: an international symposium. Trenton, NJ: Veterinary Learning Systems, 1995:28–37.

293. Jacobson ER, Brown MP, Chung M, Vliet K, Swift R. Serum concentration and disposition kinetics of gentamicin and amikacin in juvenile American alligators. J Zoo Anim Med 1988;19(4):188–94.

294. Sporle H, Gobel T, Schildger B. Blood levels of some antiinfectives in the spur-tailed tortoise (*Testudo hermanni*). Proceedings of the 4th International Colloquium Pathology and Medicine of Repiles Amphibians. Abstract.

295. Lawrence K, Needham JR, Palmer GH, Lewis JC. A preliminary study on the use of carbenicillin in snakes. J Vet Pharmacol Ther 1984;7:119–24.

296. Lawrence K, Palmer GH, Needham JR. Use of carbenicillin in two species of tortoise (*Testudo graeca and T. hermanni*). Res Vet Sci 1986;40:413–15.

297. Klingenberg RJ, Backner B. The use of ciprofloxacin, a new antibiotic in snakes. Seattle: Proceedings of the 15th International Herpetological Symposium on Captive Propagation Husbandry, 1991:127–40.

298. Lawrence K, Muggleton PW, Needham JR. Preliminary study on the use of ceftazidime, a broad spectrum cephalosporin antibiotic, in snakes. Res Vet Sci 1984;36:16–20.

299. Stamper MA, Papich M, Lewbart G, Plummer D, May S, Stoskopf M. Single dose pharmacokinetics of ceftazidime in loggerhead sea turtles (*Caretta caretta*). Proceedings of the American Association of Zoo Veterinarians, 1977:16.

300. Klingenberg RJ. Personal communication, 1994. Sheep Draw Veterinary Hospital, Greeley, CO.

301. Young LE, Schumacher J, Jacobson ER, Papich M. Disposition of enrofloxacin and its metabolite ciprofloxacin after intramuscular injection in juvenile Burmese pythons (*Python molurus bivittatus*). J Zoo Wildl Med 1997;28(1):71.

302. Prezant RM, Isaza R, Jacobson ER. Plasma concentrations and disposition kinetics of enrofloxacin in gopher tortoises (*Gopherus polyphemus*). J Zoo Wildl Med 1994;25(1):82–7.

303. Raphael BL, Papich M, Cook RA. Pharmocokinetics of enrofloxacin after a single intramuscular injection in Indian star tortoises (*Geochelone elegans*). J Zoo Wildl Med 1994;25(1):88–94.

304. Maxwell LK, Jacobson ER. Preliminary single-dose pharmacokinetics of enrofloxacin after oral and intramuscular administration in green iguanas (*Iguana iguana*). Proceedings of the American Association of Zoo Veterinarians, 1977:25.

305. Helmick KE, Papich MG, Vliet K.A, Bennett RA, Brown MR, Jacobson ER. Preliminary kinetics of single-dose intravenously administered enrofloxacin and oxytetracycline in the American alligator (*Alligator mississipiensis*). Proceedings of the American Association of Zoo Veterinarians, 1977:27–8.

306. Hilf M, Swanson D, Wagner R, Yu VL. A new dosing schedule for gentamicin in blood pythons (*Python curtus*): a pharmacokinetic study. Res Vet Sci 1991;50:127–30.

307. Raphael, B., Clark CH, Hudson R. Plasma concentration of gentamicin in turtles. J Zoo Anim Med 1985;16:136–9.

308. Teare JA, Wallace RS, Bush M. Pharmacology of gentamicin in the leopard frog (*Rana pipiens*). Proceedings of the American Association of Zoo Veterinarians, 1991.

309. Stoskopf MK Arnold J, Mason M. Aminoglycoside antibiotic levels in the aquatic salamander *Necturus necturus*. J Zoo Anim Med 1987;18(2–3):81–5.

310. Page DC, Mautino M, Derendorf H, Mechlinski W. Multiple-dose pharmacokinetics of ketoconazole administered orally to gopher tortoises (*Gopherus polyphemus*). J Zoo Wildl Med 1991;22(2):191–8.

311. Kolmstetter CK, Frazier D, Cox S, Ramsay EC. Metronidazole pharmacokinetics in yellow rat snakes (*Elaphe obsoleta quadrivitatta*). Proceedings of the American Association of Zoo Veterinarians, 1997:26.

312. Kolmstetter CK, Frazier D, Cox S, Ramsay EC. Pharmacokinetics of metronidazole in the green iguana (*Iguana iguana*). Bulletin of the Association of Reptilian and Amphibian Veterinarians, in press.

313. Holt PE. Drugs and dosages. In Cooper JE, Jackson OF, eds. Diseases of the reptilia, Vol. 2. London: Academic Press, 1981.

314. Boyer TH. Practitioner's guide to reptilian husbandry and care. Lakewood, CO: American Animal Hospital Association, 1993.

315. Hilf M, Swanson D, Wagner R, Yu VL. Pharmacokinetics of piperacillin in blood pythons (*Python curtus*) and in vitro evaluation of efficacy against aerobic gram-negative bacteria. J Zoo Wildl Med 1991;22(2):199–203.

316. Letcher J, Glade M. Efficacy of ivermectin as an anthelmintic in leopard frogs. J Am Vet Med Assoc 1992;200:537–8.

317. Klingenberg RJ. A comparison of fenbendazole and ivermectin for the treatment of nematode parasites in ball pythons, *Python regius*. Bull Assoc Rept Amphib Vet 1992;2(2):5–6.

318. Lawerence K. Praziquantel as a taeniacide in snakes. Vet Rec 1983;113:200.

319. Boyer D. Snake mite (*Ophionyssus natricus*) eradication utilizing permectin spray. Bull Assoc Rept Amphib Vet 1994;4(2):3.

320. Abrahams R. Ivermectin as a spray for treatment of snake mites. Bull Assoc Rept Amphib Vet 1992;2(1):8.

321. Mader DR. Personal communication, 1994. Long Beach Animal Hospital, Long Beach, CA.

322. Boyer TH. Metabolic bone disease. Hypovitaminosis A. In Mader DR, ed. Reptile medicine and surgery. Philadelphia: W.B. Saunders, 1995:382–92.

323. Mader DR. Use of calcitonin in green iguanas, *Iguana iguana*, with metabolic bone disease. Bull Assoc Rept Amphib Vets 1993;3(1):5.

324. Barten SL. Oviductal rupture in a Burmese python (*Python molorus bivittatus*) treated with oxytocin for egg retention. J Zoo Anim Med 1985;16:141–3.

325. Lloyd M.Vasotocin—the reptilian alternative to oxytocin? Bull Assoc Rept Amphib Vet 1992;2(1):5.

326. Boyer TH. Clinical anesthesia of reptiles. Bull Assoc Rept Amphib Vet 1992;2(2):10–13.

327. Millichamp N. Surgical techniques in reptiles. In Jacobson E, Kollias G Jr, eds. Exotic animals. New York: Churchill Livingstone, 1988:49–59.

328. Johnson J. Anesthesia, analgesia, and euthanasia of reptiles and amphibians. Proceedings of the American Association of Zoo Veterinarians, 1991:132–8.

329. Barten SL. Personal communication, 1994. Vernon Hills Animal Hospital, Mundelein, IL.

330. Bennett RA. A review of anesthesia and chemical restraint in reptiles. J Zoo Wildlife Med 1991;22:282–303.

331. Divers SJ. The use of propofol in reptile anesthesia. Assoc Reptilian Amphibian Vets Proc 1996: 57-59.

332. Burghardt GM, Stanley Rand G. Iguanas of the world: their behavior, ecology, and conservation. Park Ridge NJ: Noyes Publishing, 1982.

333. Bennett RA, Schumacher J, Hedjazi-Haring K, Newell SM. Cardiopulmonary and anesthetic affects of propofol administered intra-osseously in green iguanas. J Am Vet Med Assoc 1998; 212(1):93.

334. Speroni JA, Soraci A, Giambeluca L, Errecalde JO. Farmacocinetica de cefoperazona tras su administracion intramuscular a *Hydrodynastes gigas* (Ophidia, Colubridae). Beunos Aires, Argentina: AHA Communications Meeting, 1989.

335. Speroni JA, Soraci A, Giambeluca L, Errecalde JO. Farmacocinetica de cefoperazona tras su administracion intramuscular a *Tupinambis teguixin* (Sauria, Teidae). Beunos Aires, Argentina;: AHA Communications Meeting, 1989.

Figures

Figure 1 Severe thermal burns in *Chamaeleo calyptratus* from a 250-watt spot light 6 inches above basking area.

Figure 2 Chalk line development visible in leopard tortoise egg, *Geochelone pardalis*, about 1 month into development. The chalk line starts dorsally and then spreads ventrally in fertile eggs; infertile eggs remain fairly lucent.

Figure 3 Hatchling leopard tortoise, *G. pardalis*, on first day after emerging from the egg. Note the large normal yolk sac.

Figure 4 Same hatchling as in figure 3 on the second day after egg emergence. The yolk sac has been absorbed into the coelom.

Figure 5 Same hatchling on the ninth day after emergence. The umbilical plastral defect is almost totally closed.

Figure 6 Severe dog gnaw trauma in an ornate box turtle, *Terrapene ornata ornata*.

Figure 7 Male (left) and female three-toed box turtles, *Terrapene carolina, triungius*. Note the longer tail of the male with the cloacal opening caudal to the dorsal carapace. *Courtesy of Colorado State University, Veterinary Teaching Hospital.*

Figure 8 Male box turtles have brighter colored irises than females.

Figure 9 Female box turtles often have reddish brown to yellow irises.

Figure 10 The humeral plexus is a good site for repeated phlebotomy.

Figure 11 The jugular is more prominent than normal in this three-toed box turtle. The jugular vein is a common venipuncture site.

Figure 12 Early vitamin A deficiency in a three-toed box turtle, *Terrapene carolina triungius.* Note the blepharoedema.

Figure 13 Iatrogenic hypervitaminosis A in a three-toed box turtle, *Terrapene carolina triungius.* Notice the sloughing epidermis on the right leg.

Figure 14 Nasal discharge in a yellow foot tortoise, *Geochelone denticulata.* Nasal discharge is always abnormal in turtles.

Figure 15 Red-eared slider, *Trachemys scripta elegans*, unable to float levelly, which is often suggestive of lower respiratory tract disease.

Figure 16 Middle ear abscess in a three-toed box turtle, *Terrapene carolina triungius.*

Figure 17 Bot fly cyst in an ornate box turtle, *Terrapin o. ornata.* Note the black-rimmed opening that the larvae breathe through. Several larvae are found per cyst, and several cysts per turtle are typical.
Courtesy of Colorado State University, Veterinary Teaching Hospital.

Figure 18 Cystic calculi in desert tortoise, *Gopherus agassizii.* The larger size of the right liver lobe relative to the left is thought to be the reason for the predominance of stones in the left lobe of the bladder.
Courtesy of Colorado State University, Veterinary Teaching Hospital.

Figure 19	Prolapsed penis in a Hermann's tortoise, *Testudo hermanni*, secondary to metabolic bone disease. *Courtesy of Colorado State University, Veterinary Teaching Hospital.*
Figure 20	Two-year-old ornate box turtle with metabolic bone disease. The shell was soft, but also see the upturned marginals, posteriorly curved anterior rhamphotheca, and increased vertical growth in bridge area.
Figure 21	Pyramidal shell growth in a spurred tortoises, *Geochelone sulcata*, fed primarily monkey chow biscuits. *Courtesy of Colorado State University, Veterinary Teaching Hospital.*
Figure 22	Ventral femoral pores in a male (left) and female green iguana, *Iguana iguana*. Femoral pores are not easily distinguishable until iguanas reach sexual maturity.
Figure 23	Young green iguanas, *Iguana iguana*, are easily probed with small snake probes. Males probe more than twice the depth of females; this example is a male.
Figure 24	Cagemate trauma in a young green iguana, *Iguana iguana*. Iguanas do best if housed individually unless very large cages are available.
Figure 25	Hot rock burns on the ventrum of a green iguana, *Iguana iguana*. Owners often report that their iguana spends an inordinate amount of time basking on the hot rock; this indicates that the ambient temperatures is too cool. Hot rocks are not a preferred method of providing heat.
Figure 26	Lateral radiographs for green iguanas are easiest if the wrists are taped together and the knees taped to the tail. A wooden spoon can push the arms out of coelomic picture. Iguanas relax well in this position and good lateral alignment is obtained.

Figure 27 Lateral radiograph of iguana with acute coelomic distress and bloating. The cecum is displaced dorsally and anteriorly (just posterior to the lungs) and an increased gas pattern is visible in the colon. At exploratory celiotomy a 360 cecal volvulus was found.

Figure 28 The medial tibial crest is an easy area in which to insert an intraosseous 20- to 22-gauge needle under local or general anesthesia. Iguanas tolerate this quite well; continuous fluid administration is easiest with a pump.

Figure 29 Syringe cases make excellent mouth speculums for lizards. Oral medications and stomach tubes are easily administered through the speculum.
Courtesy of Colorado State University, Veterinary Teaching Hospital.

Figure 30 Normal iguanas should lift their entire body and proximal tail up off the ground when threatened or while walking (compare with next figure).

Figure 31 Iguanas with metabolic bone disease are often unable to lift their pelvis or tail up off the ground.

Figure 32 Flap-necked chameleon, *Chamaeleo dilepsis*, raised on unsupplemented crickets and mealworms. Most bones were soft and pliable; the tibiotarsus is obviously fractured. Insects are calcium deficient unless properly fed and dusted.

Figure 33 Metabolic bone disease in a green iguana, *Iguana iguana*. Note the overall decreased opacity to bone making the pelvis and transverse vertebral processes difficult to distinguish from soft tissue. Fractures and fibrous osteodystrophy are present in the distal tibiotarsi.
Courtesy of Colorado State University, Veterinary Teaching Hospital.

Figure 34 Normal bone opacity of a chuckawalla, *Sauromalus obesus*, except for osteomyelitis in swollen foot. Note that the pelvis and transverse vertebral processes are both easily visualized and the typical lytic nature of osteomyelitis. Compare with figure 33. *Courtesy of Colorado State University, Veterinary Teaching Hospital.*

Figure 35 Renomegaly is easily observed in this green iguana, under the lumbar musculature just anterior and dorsal to the pelvis.

Figure 36 Long tapered feces from an iguana with renomegaly. Feces are thinned as the colon passes between the enlarged kidneys.

Figure 37 Renomegaly in an iguana, *Iguana iguana*, that died of renal failure. Notice the barely visible colon coursing thorough the kidneys.

Figure 38 Cystic calculi in a green iguana; the ventral outline of the radiolucent cecum is also visible.

Figure 39 Idiopathic bloat in a young green iguana, *Iguana iguana*.

Figure 40 Exposure gingivitis is common in green iguanas if the upper and lower jaws are slightly misaligned. Past metabolic bone disease often predisposes iguanas to exposure gingivitis.

Figure 41 Rostral abscess in a green iguana. Even large abscesses such as this respond well to treatment.

Figure 42 Epidermal inclusion cyst on the dorsal tail of a green iguana.

Figure 43 Gravid female iguana; eggs or follicles are bulging from the caudal coelomic wall. Little wonder that gravid females are anorexic.

Figure 44	Lateral radiograph of eggs in the oviduct of a green iguana. Note that distinct egg shapes are visible and the eggs appear much less bunched up than preovulatory follicles.
Figure 45	Egg yolk coelomitis in a dead green iguana. The ovaries should also be removed in lizards if the gravid oviducts are removed.
Figure 46	Multifocal skin necrosis in a green iguana secondary to heavy mite infestations.
Figure 47	Red mites are visible up under the scales on the front foot of this green iguana. Mites are difficult to see grossly until present in large numbers.
Figure 48	Hemipenal waxy casts protruding from the cloaca of a male green iguana. Waxy casts can be carefully pulled out while everting the hemipenes. Often these casts are palpable but not protruding from the cloaca.
Figure 49	Severe rat bite trauma in this *Boa constrictor* eventually resulted in the snake's demise. Rodents should never be left hungry and unattended with reptiles.
Figure 50	Stuck shed, dysecdysis, in a *Boa constrictor*. Note the gaping mouth, wrinkled skin, and severe appearance.
Figure 51	Same snake as in figure 50 after soaking in shallow water overnight with a rock. The snake shed cleanly on its own and is back to normal.
Figure 52	Retained spectacle in a Burmese python, *Python molorus bivittatus*. Retained spectacles are easily removed with Q-tips, fine tweezers, or one's fingers. Note the retained shed skin periorbitally.
Figure 53	Spectacular corneal damage in a ball python, *Python regius*, resulting from overzealous attempts at removing a suspected retained spectacle.

Figure 54 Snake mites are often visible between the gular scales, as in this Burmese python.

Figure 55 Wooden Q-tips act as good disposable mouth speculums for snakes. Light pressure against the inner maxillary tooth rows elicits a gape response.

Figure 56 Caseous cellular debris, swollen gingiva and anterior maxillae, petechiae, and thick mucus are typical for infectious stomatitis.
Courtesy of Elliott Jacobson, DVM, PhD, DACZM.

Figure 57 Green anaconda, *Eunectes murinus*, illustrating the epaxial grooves. Notice that the epaxial grooves are filled out in the rear half of this snake, indicating that it has good body weight.

Figure 58 Everting or "popping" the hemipenes in a ball python, *Python regius*. This is an easy method of sexing young snakes, but if the hemipenes fail to evert, sex is inconclusive (which can be frustrating). This procedure becomes harder to do as the snake gets larger.

Figure 59 Cardiocentesis is the preferred method of blood collection in boids. Note that the heart is pushed to the side and forward to stabilize it, while a second person secures the heart anteriorly. Anesthesia makes the procedure easier for all parties, especially with larger snakes.
Courtesy of Colorado State University, Veterinary Teaching Hospital.

Figure 60 Severe respiratory distress in a ball python, *Python regius*. Not only is the snake opening its mouth to breathe, but also the head and neck are elevated to ease tracheal air passage.

Figure 61 Opisthotonus or corkscrewing in a Burmese python with inclusion body disease virus.

Figure 62 Eastern black king snake, *Lampropeltus getulus niger*, that is egg bound. Several egg outlines are visible; ovocentesis of the caudalmost egg often permits ovipositon.

Figure 63 Small white plaques on the head of a spectacled caiman, *Caiman crocodilus*, from caiman pox.

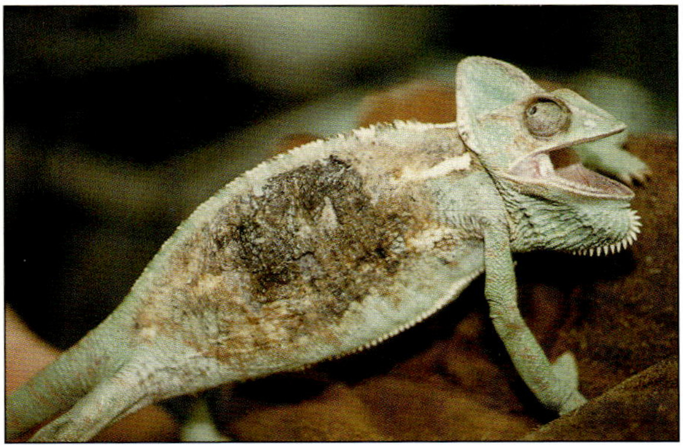

Figure 1

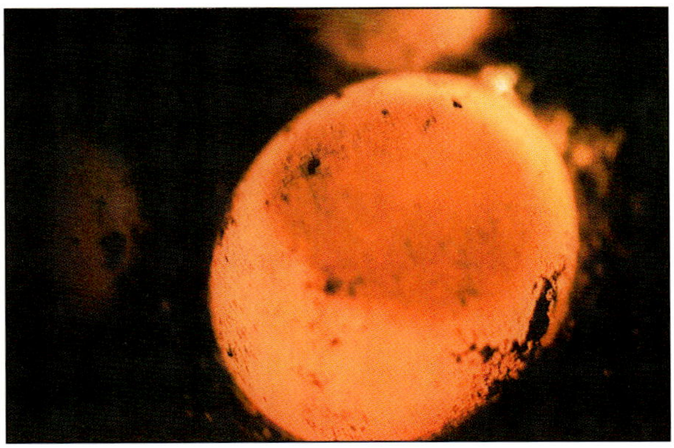

Figure 2

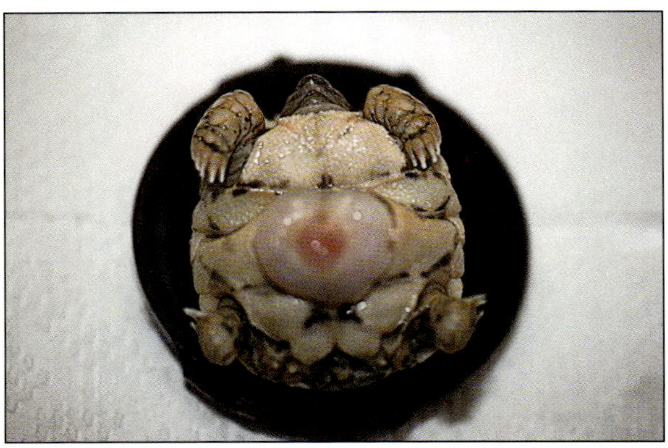

Figure 3

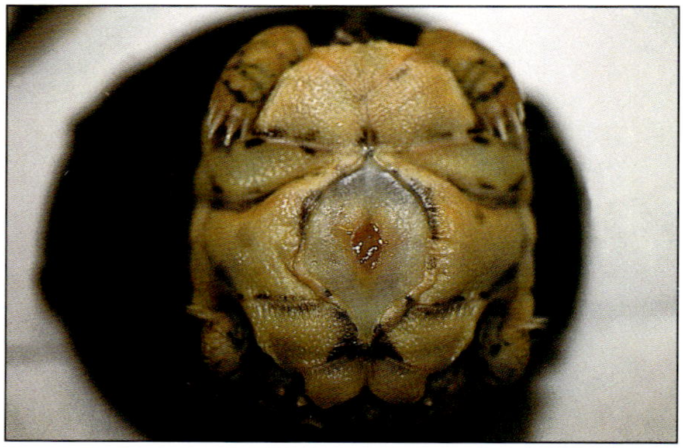

Figure 4

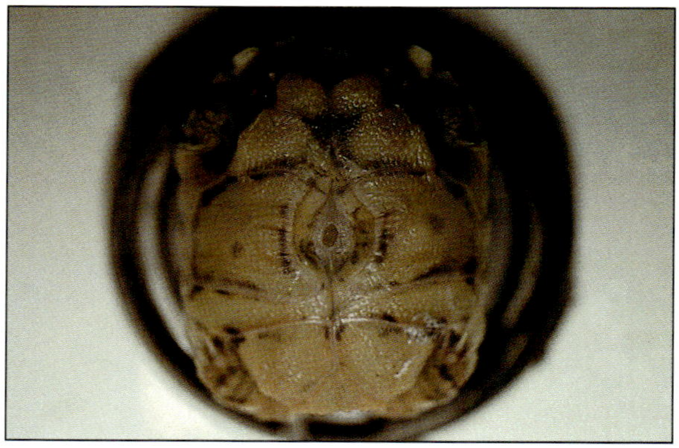

Figure 5

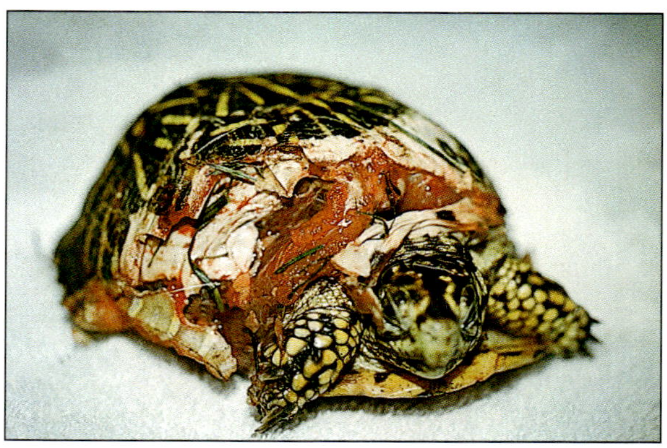

Figure 6

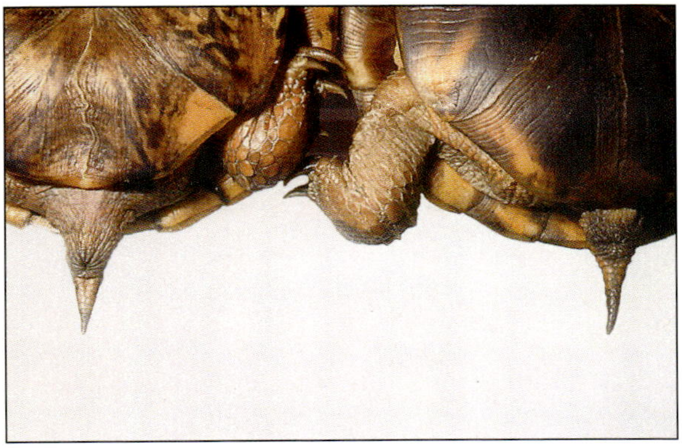

Figure 7

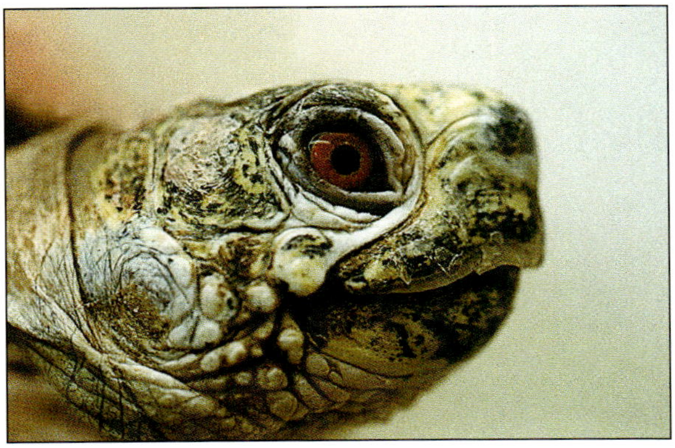

Figure 8

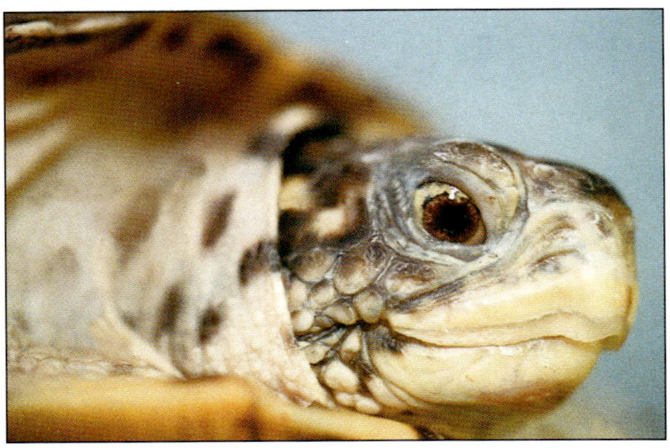

Figure 9

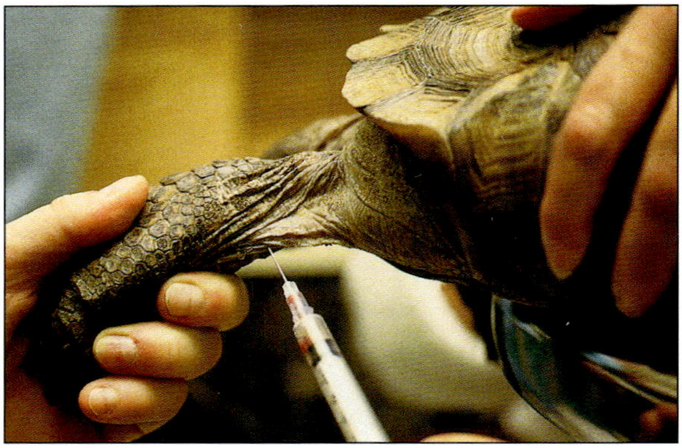

Figure 10

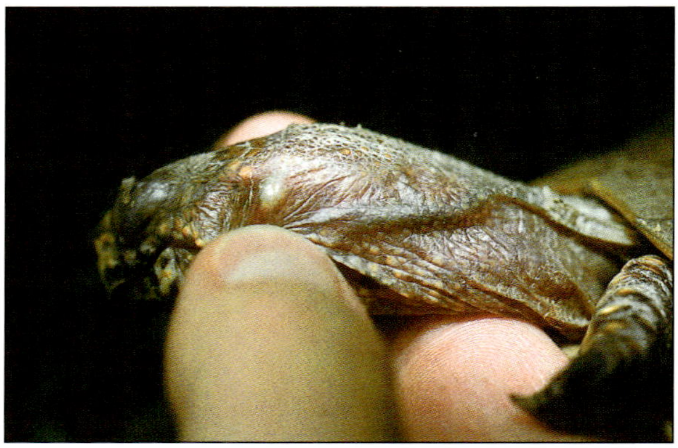

Figure 11

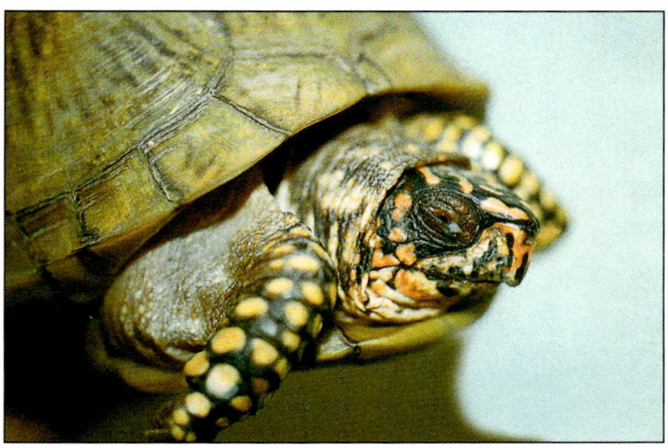

Figure 12

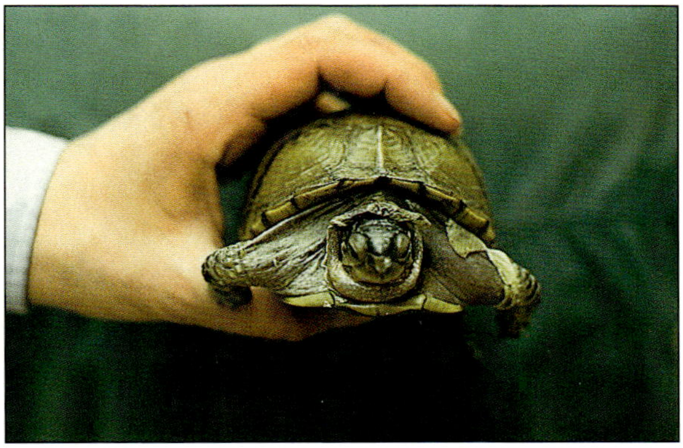

Figure 13

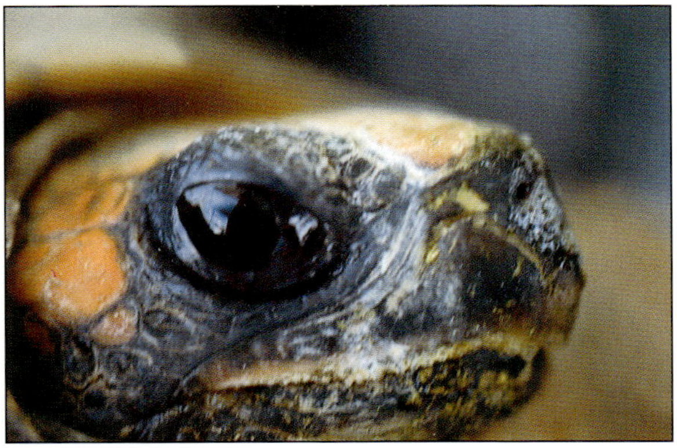

Figure 14

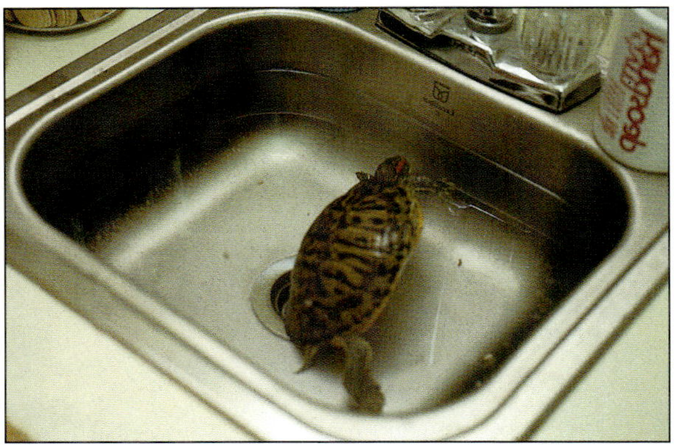

Figure 15

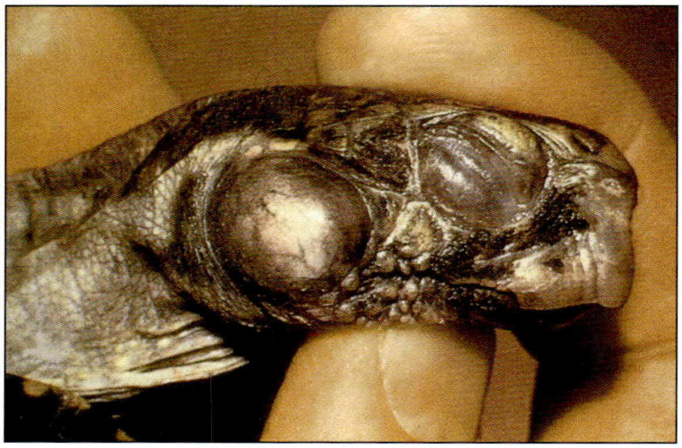

Figure 16

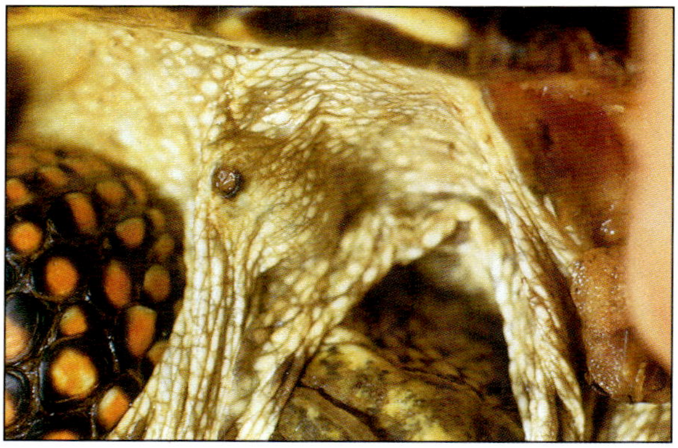

Figure 17

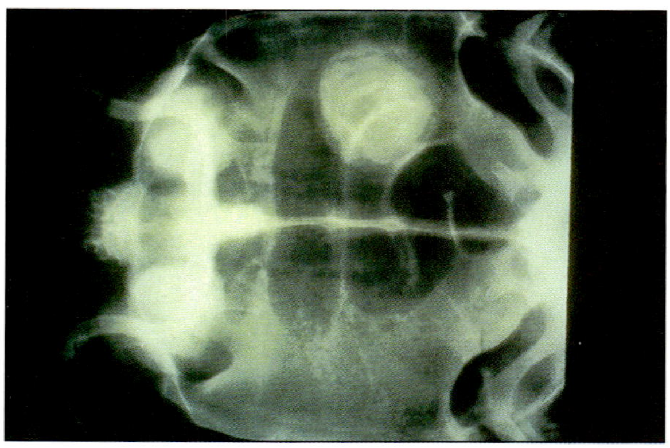

Figure 18

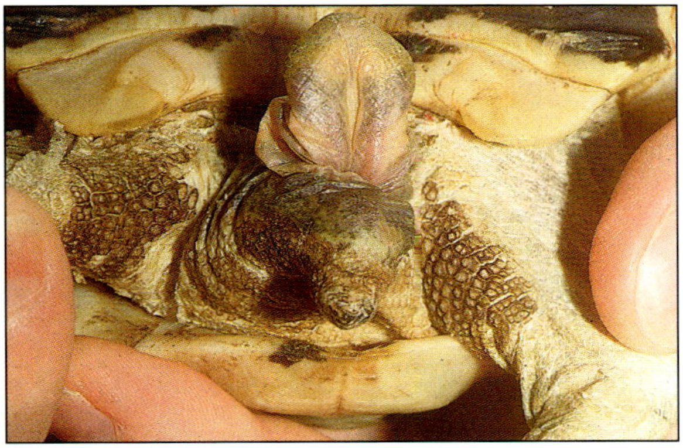

Figure 19

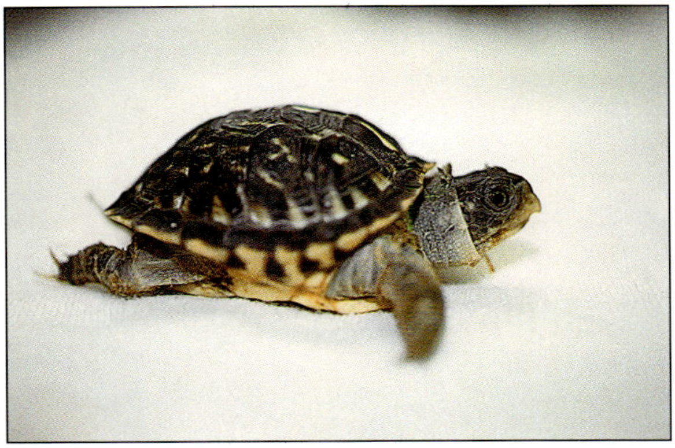

Figure 20

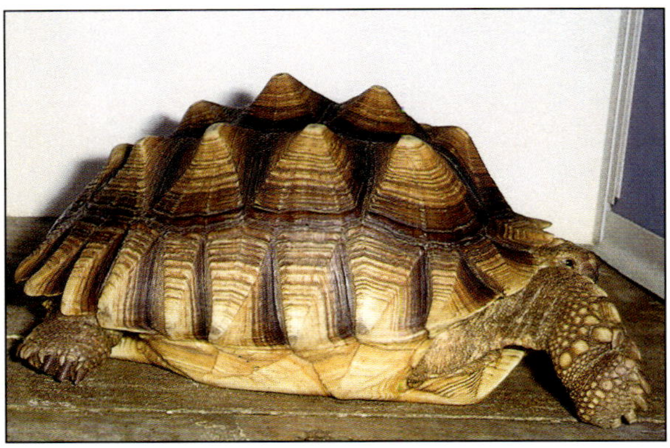

Figure 21

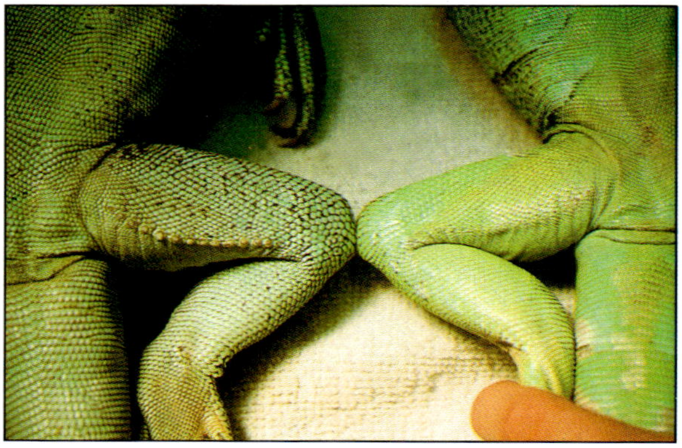

Figure 22

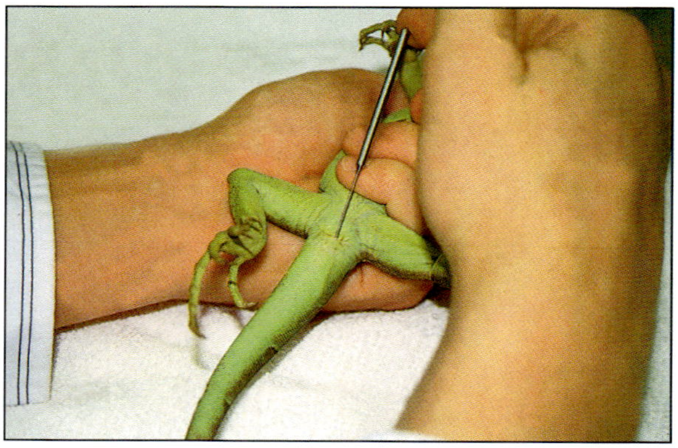

Figure 23

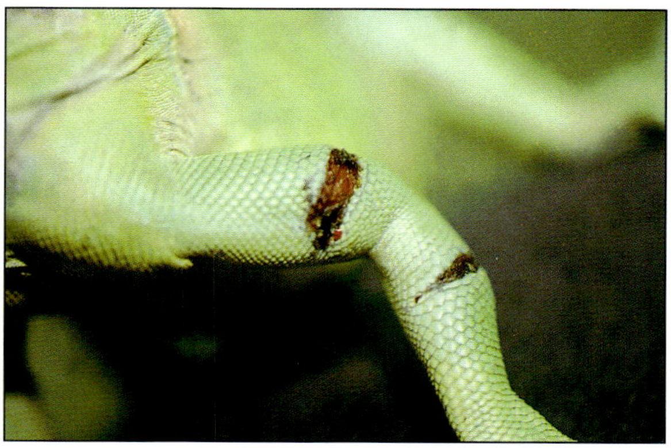

Figure 24

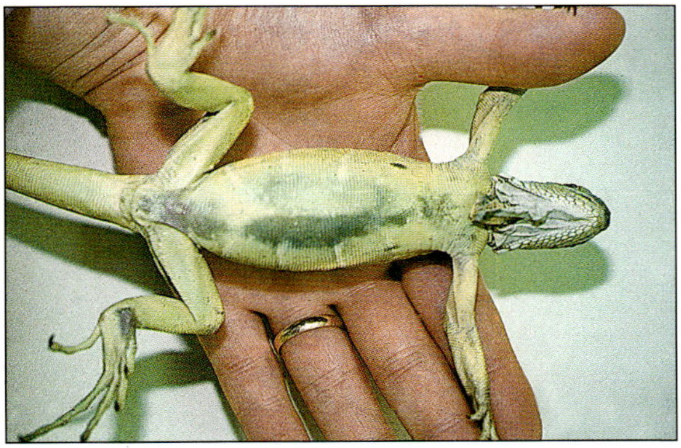

Figure 25

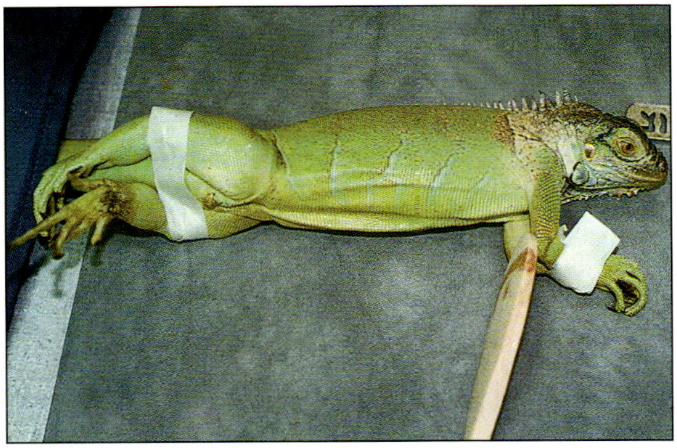

Figure 26

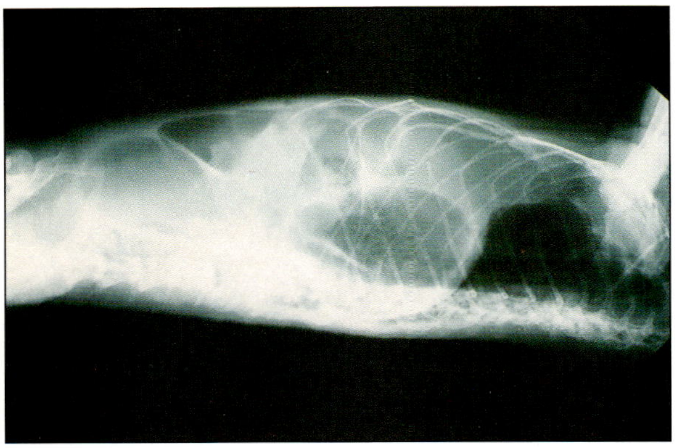

Figure 27

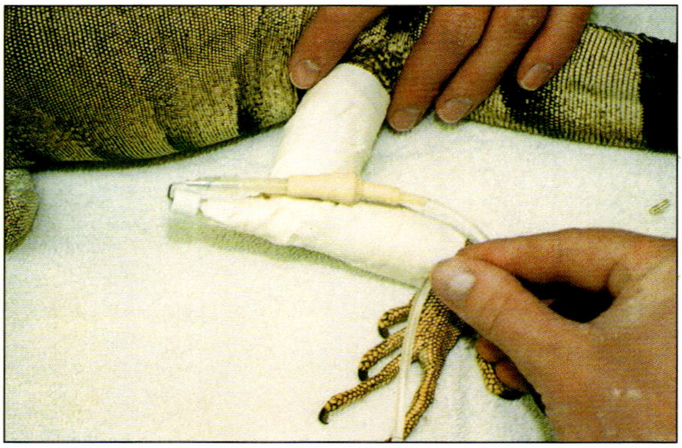

Figure 28

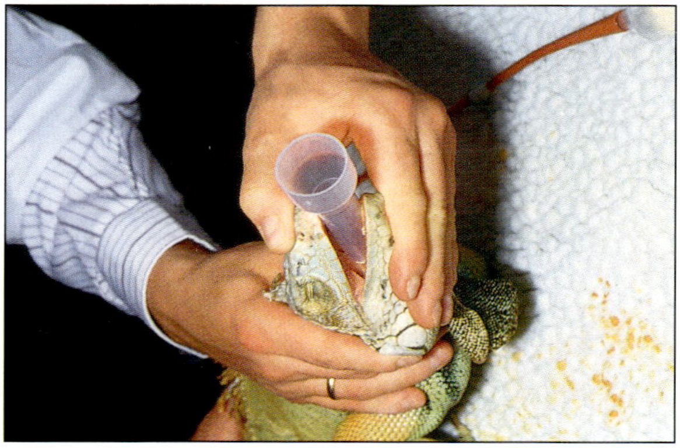

Figure 29

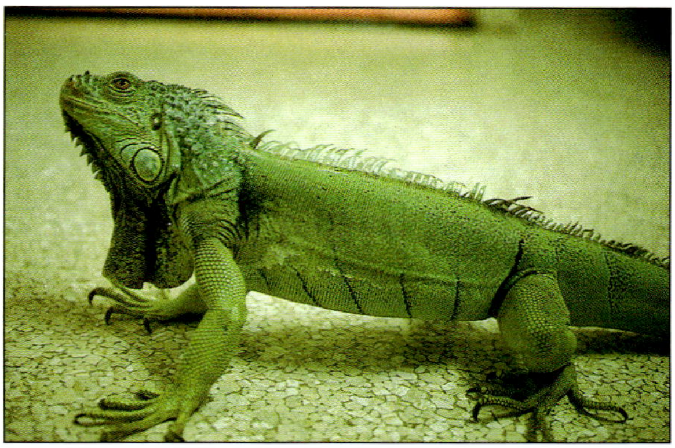

Figure 30

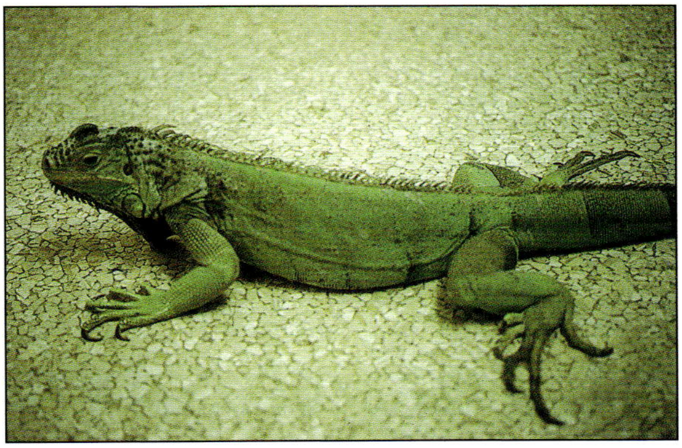

Figure 31

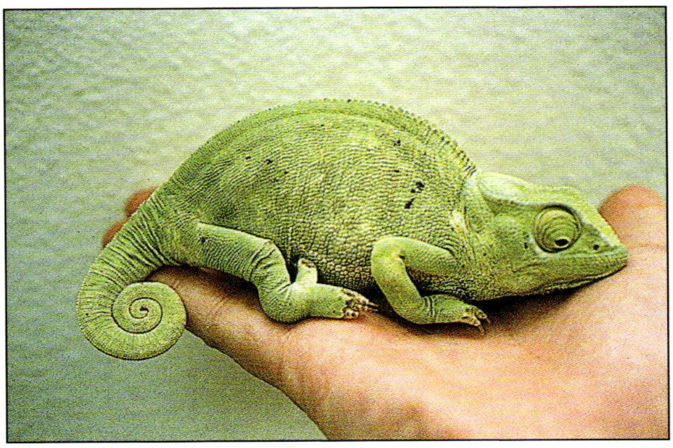

Figure 32

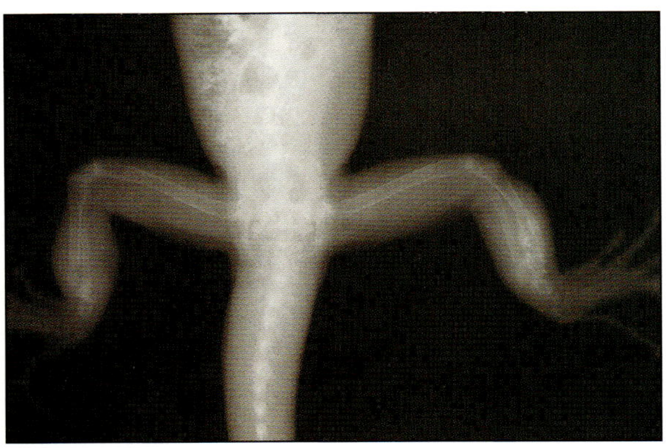

Figure 33

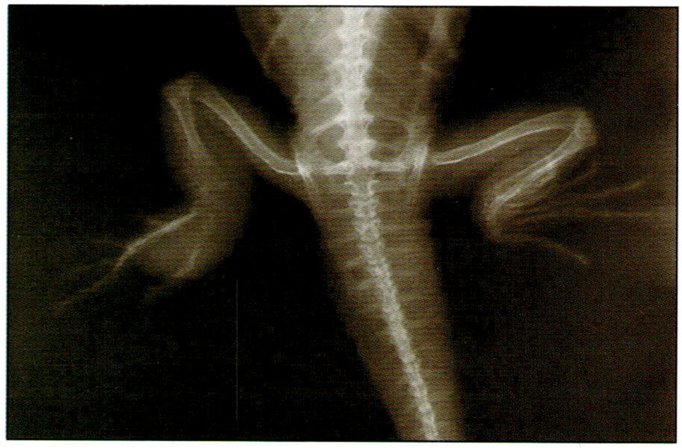

Figure 34

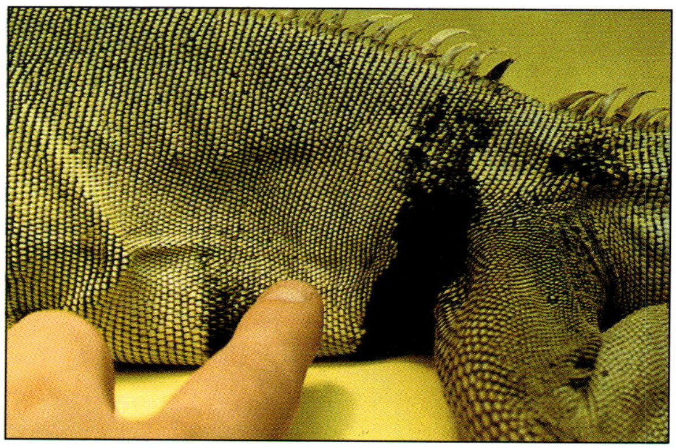

Figure 35

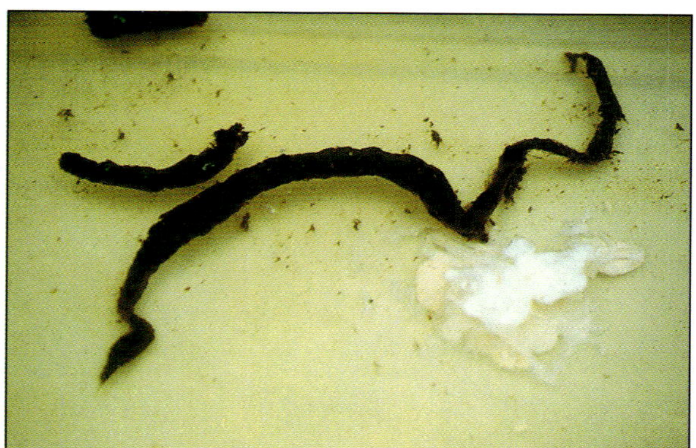

Figure 36

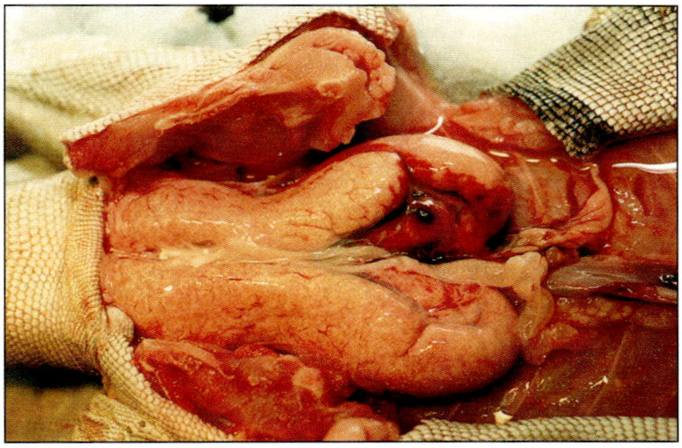

Figure 37

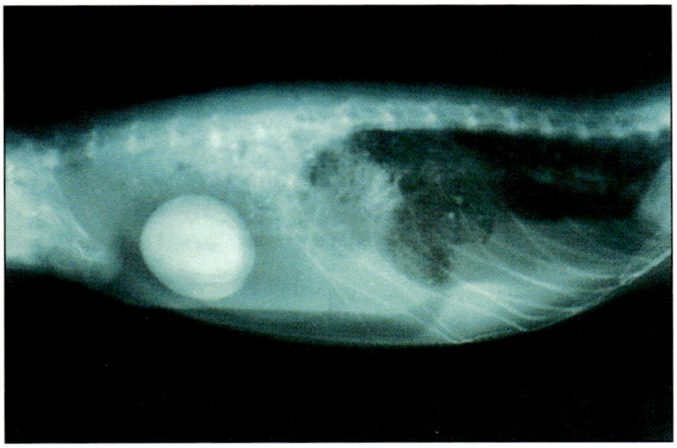

Figure 38

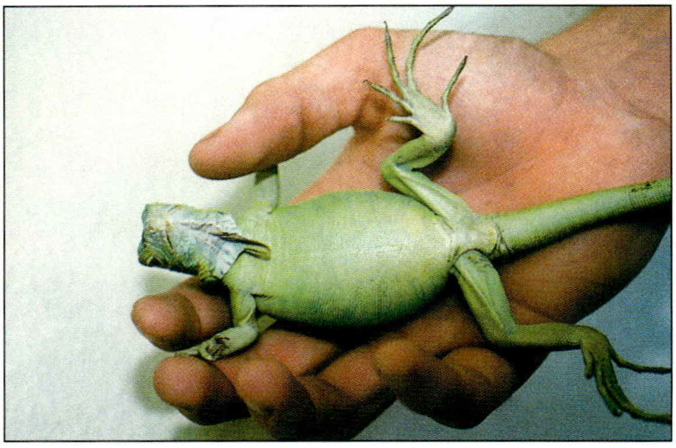

Figure 39

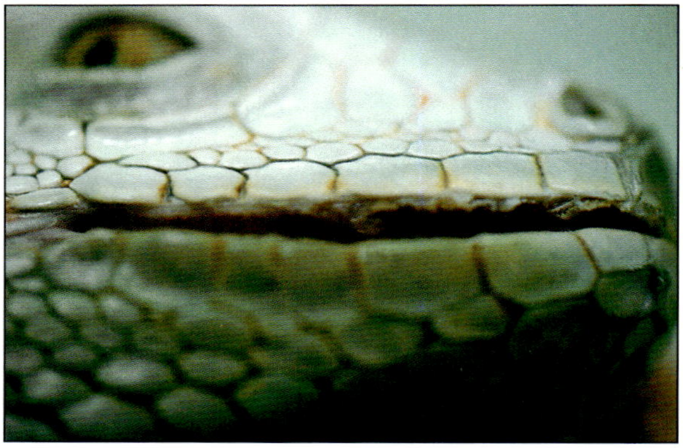

Figure 40

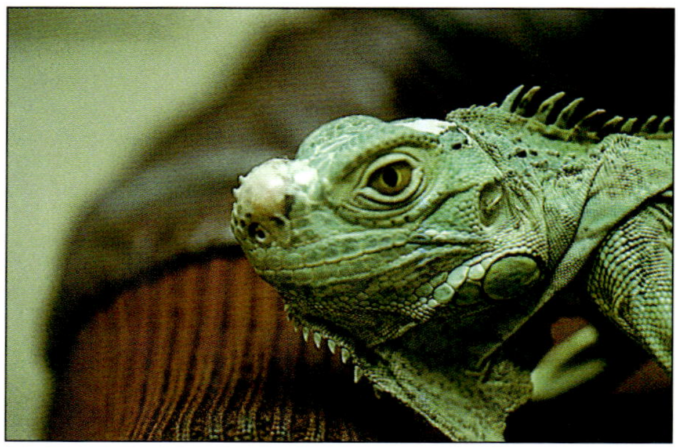

Figure 41

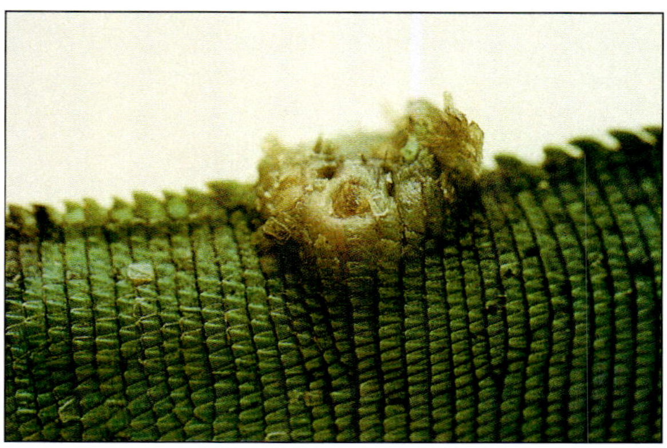

Figure 42

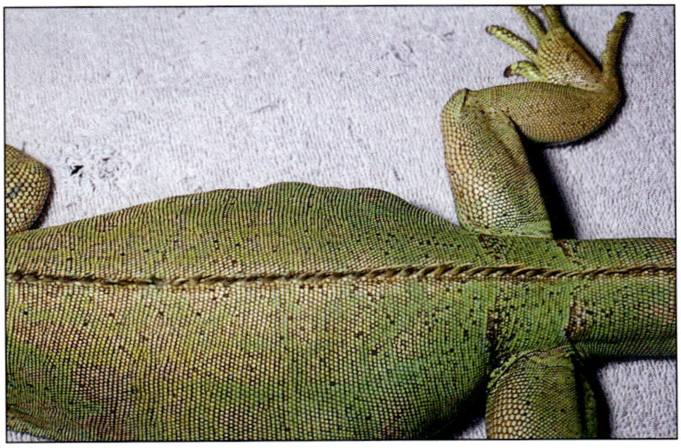

Figure 43

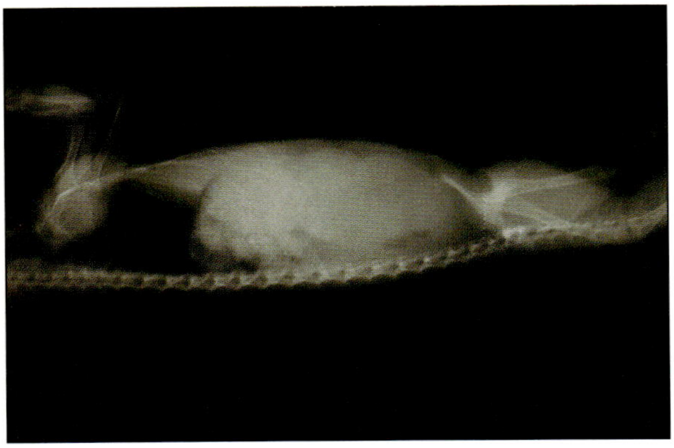

Figure 44

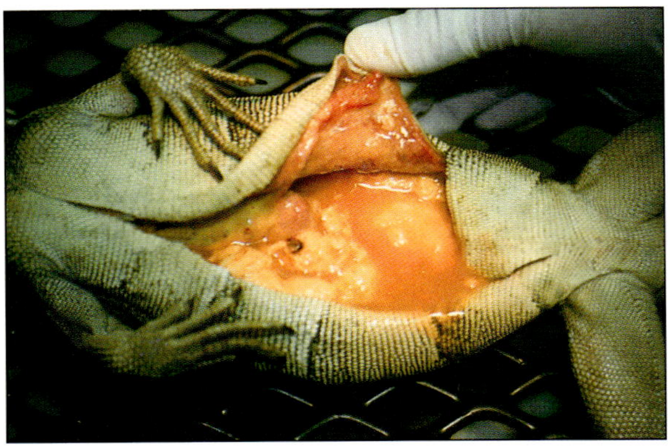

Figure 45

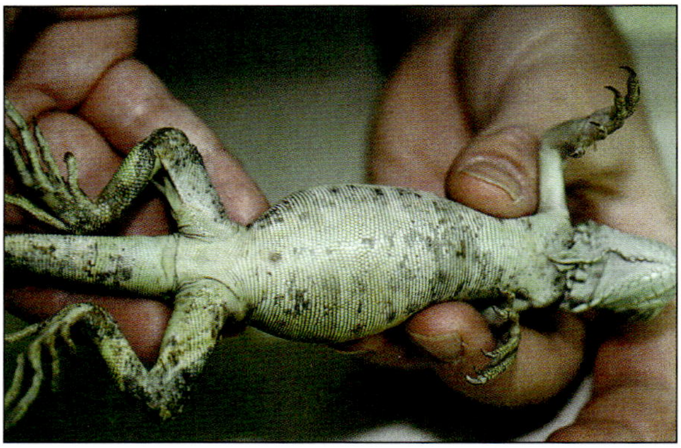

Figure 46

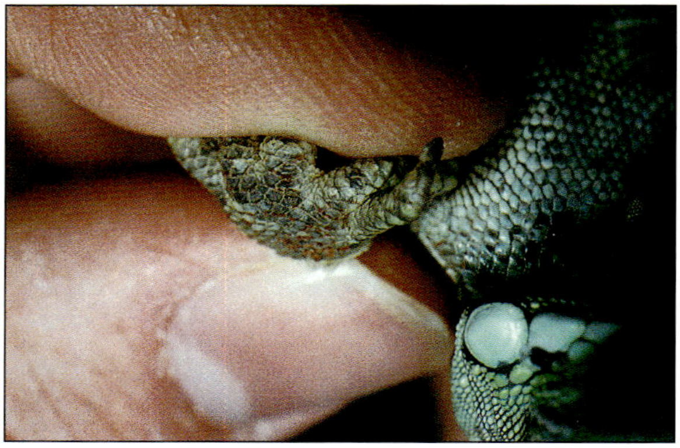

Figure 47

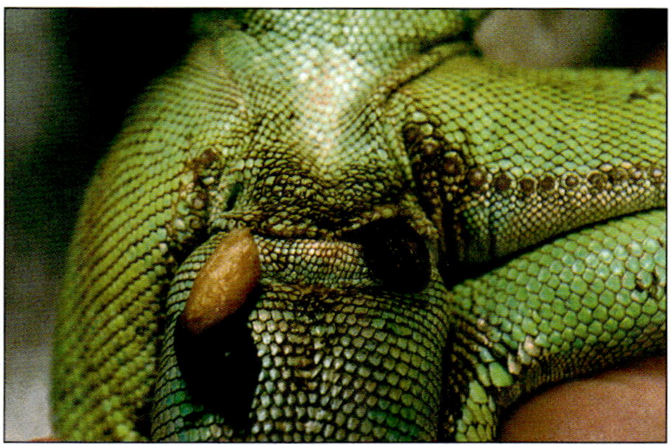

Figure 48

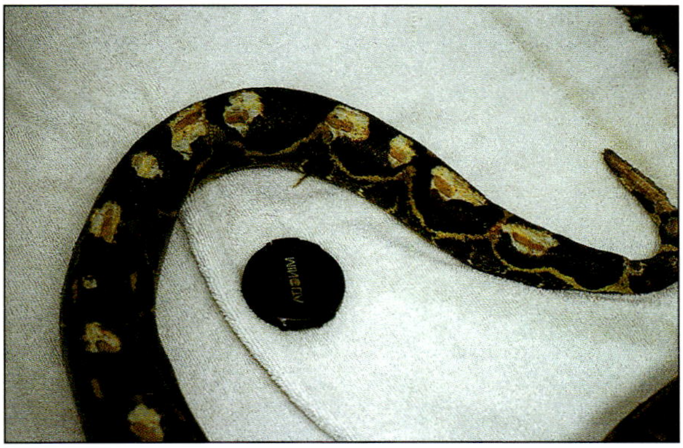

Figure 49

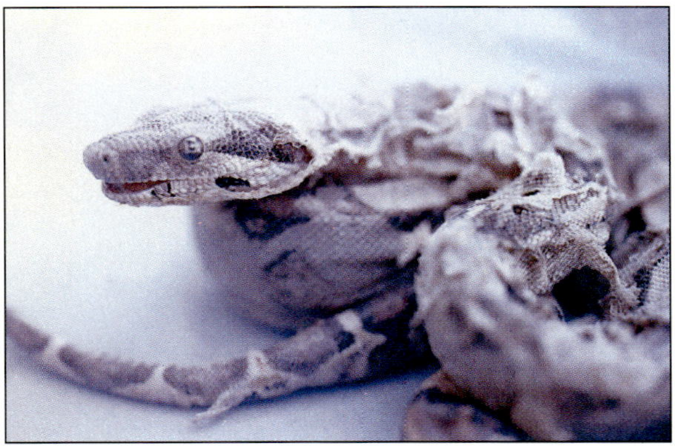

Figure 50

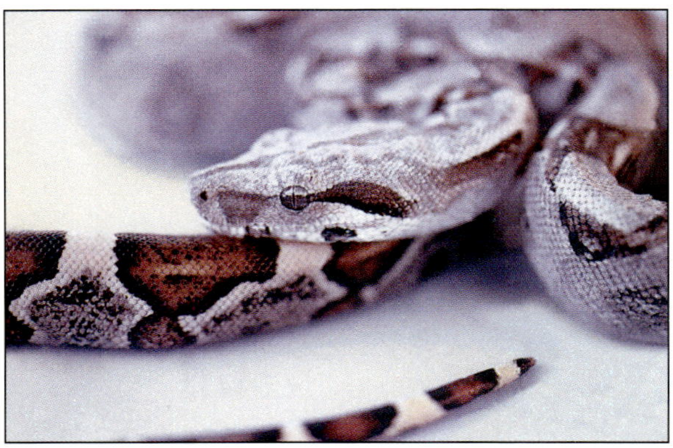

Figure 51

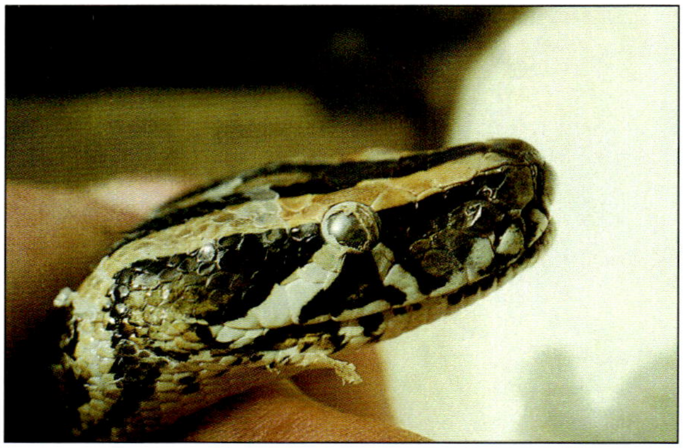

Figure 52

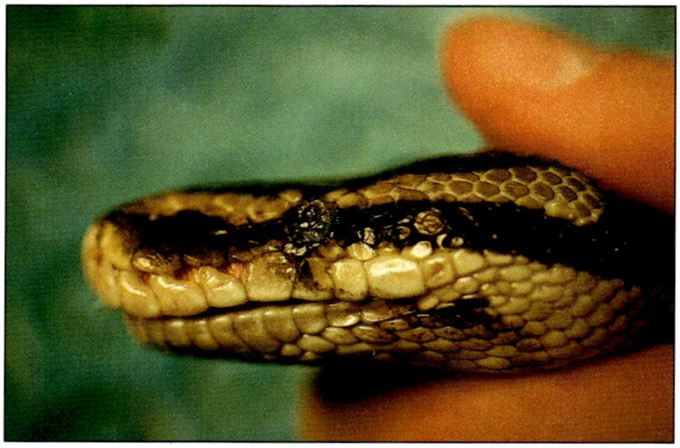

Figure 53

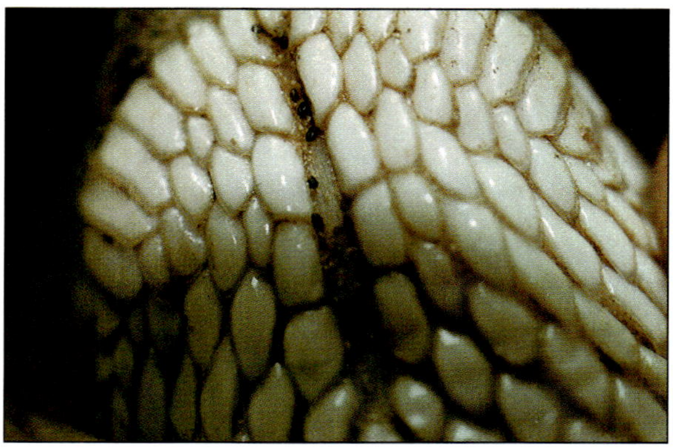

Figure 54

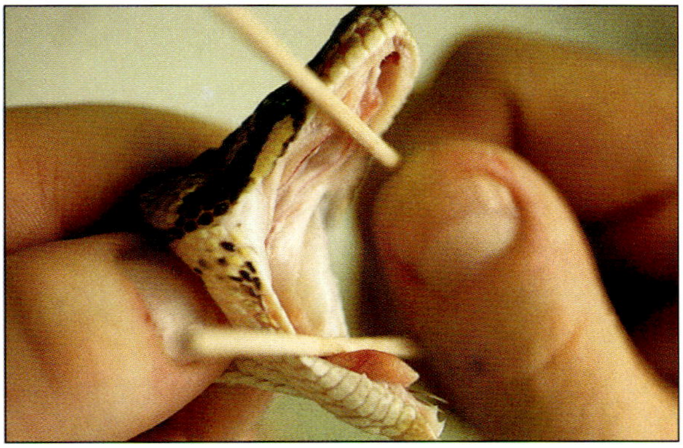

Figure 55

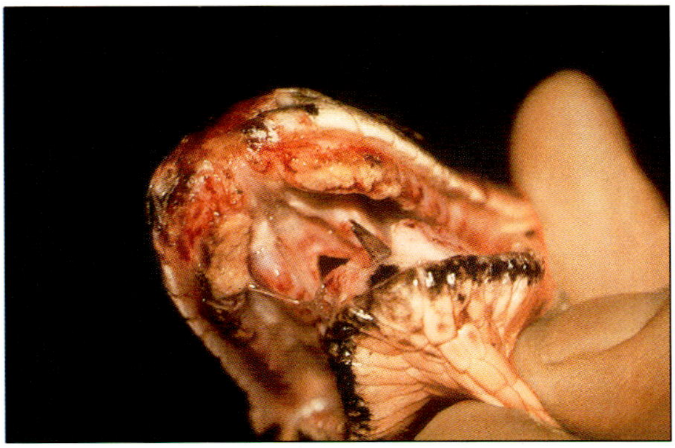

Figure 56

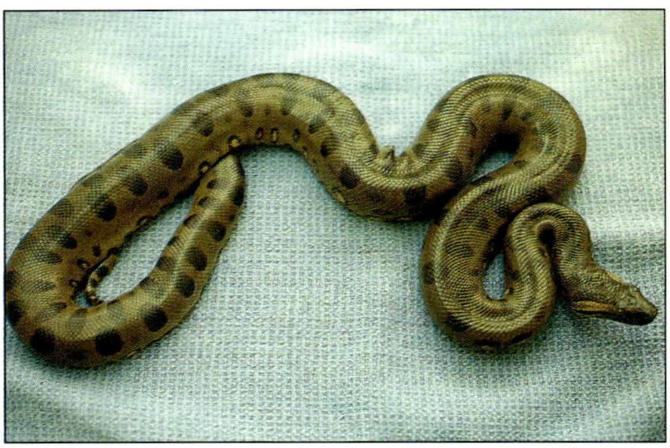

Figure 57

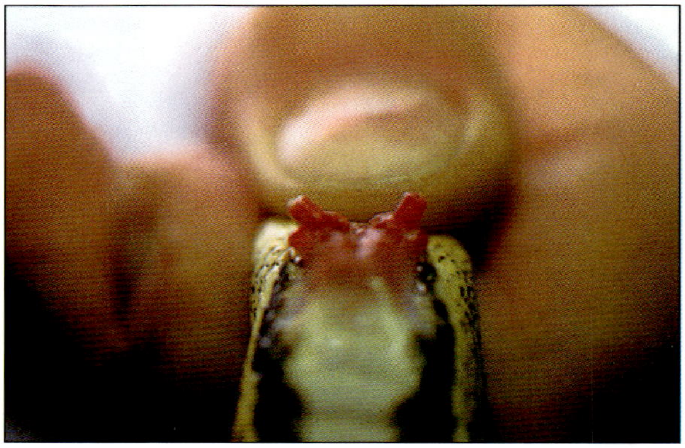

Figure 58

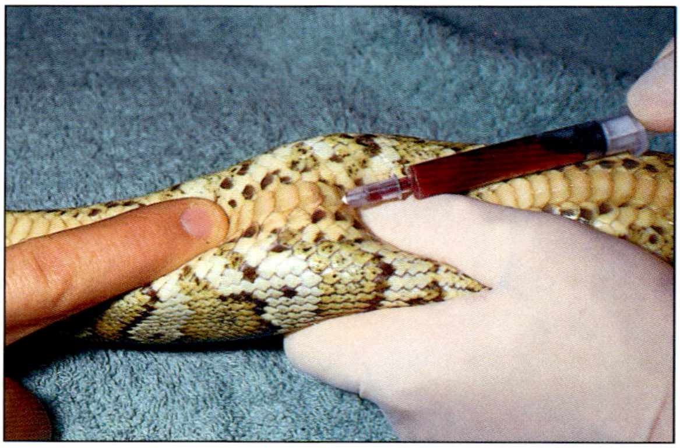

Figure 59

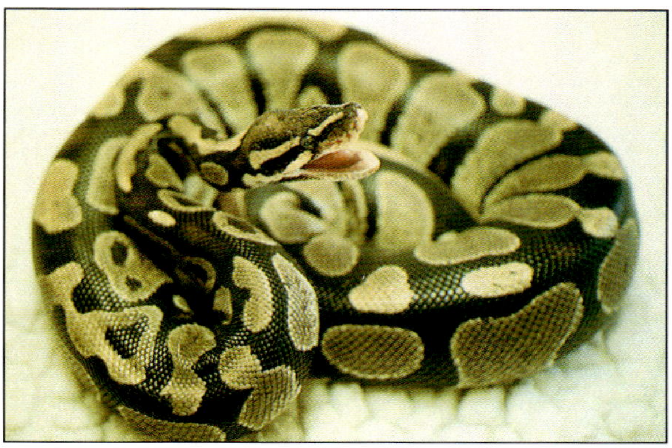

Figure 60

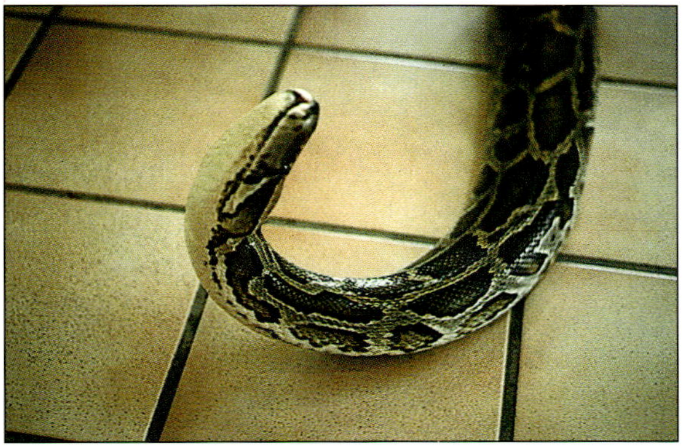

Figure 61

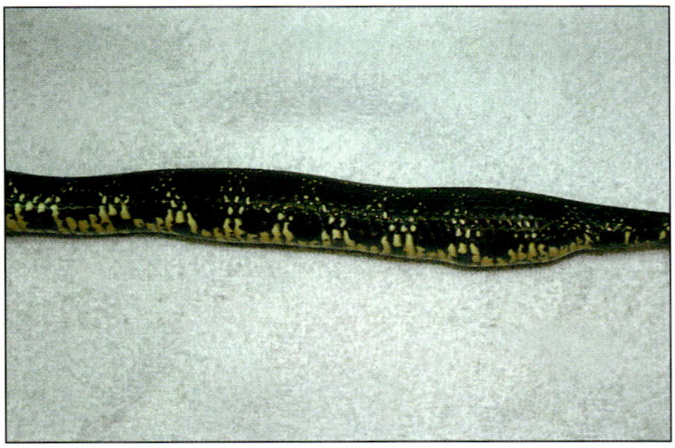

Figure 62

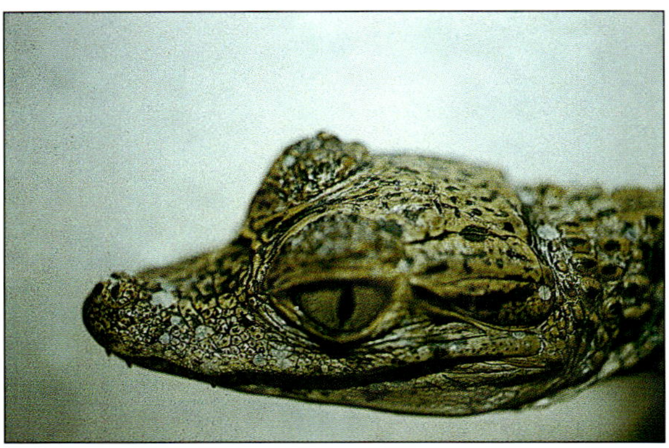

Figure 63

Index

NOTE: f. refers to figure legend, t. to table.

Index

Notes

Notes

About the Author

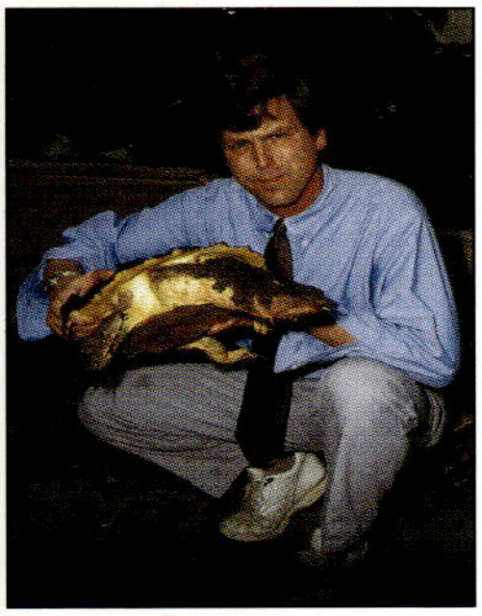

Dr. Thomas H. Boyer has had a life-long fascination with reptiles. After graduating from veterinary school in 1989, Dr. Boyer pursued an active interest in veterinary care of reptiles. In 1991 he co-founded the Association of Reptilian and Amphibian Veterinarians (ARAV). He created the Bulletin of the ARAV and has served as editor since its inception. The American Animal Hospital Association published the first edition of his book, *A Practitioner's Guide to Reptilian Husbandry and Care*, in 1993. Dr. Boyer spent 1995 as a clinical instructor in exotic animal medicine at the Colorado State University School of Veterinary Medicine and Biomedical Sciences. Dr. Boyer has produced over 100 articles, chapters, and lectures on diseases and care of reptiles. He lives with his wife, Lilia; two daughters, Ariel and Tara; and assorted reptiles and pets in sunny, subtropical San Diego.